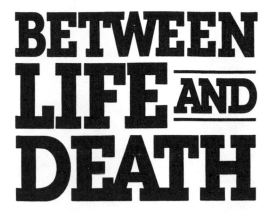

BETWEEN LIFE AND DEATH

The Life-Support Dilemma

KENNETH E. SCHEMMER, M.D.
with Dave and Neta Jackson

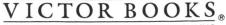

VICTOR BOOKS®

A DIVISION OF SCRIPTURE PRESS PUBLICATIONS INC.
USA CANADA ENGLAND

Scripture references, unless otherwise noted, are from the *Holy Bible New International Version,* © 1973, 1978, 1984, International Bible Society. Used by permission of Zondervan Bible Publishers. Quotations marked TLB are taken from *The Living Bible,* © 1971, Tyndale House Publishers, Wheaton, IL 60189. Used by permission. Quotations marked NKJV are from *The New King James Version,* © 1979, 1980, 1982, Thomas Nelson, Inc., Publishers.

Recommended Dewey Decimal Classification: 241
Suggested Subject Heading: CHRISTIAN ETHICS—MEDICAL

Library of Congress Catalog Card Number: 88-62850
ISBN: 0-89693-684-8

To Mansell Pattison, M.D., a friend who has taught me much about caring for the dying, wrote for me the foreword to Between Faith and Tears, *and who is himself, at the writing of this book, sustained by a life-support system.*

ACKNOWLEDGEMENTS

I wish to acknowledge the work of four professors who, through their writings and conferences, have molded my approach to the care of patients who are dying, particularly as reflected by their cited contributions in this book:

E. Mansell Pattison, M.D., chairman, department of psychiatry at the Medical College of Georgia, Augusta.

Edwin Sheidman, Ph.D., professor of thanatology at the UCLA School of Medicine, Los Angeles.

Marvin Krant, M.D., professor of psychiatry, Harvard Medical School, Boston.

Robert Jay Lifton, distinguished professor of psychiatry and psychology at John Jay College and The Graduate Center of the City University of New York.

Richard Glasgow, legal counsel to the Register of Copyrights, United States Government, a personal friend and trusted Christian confidant whose deep insight into the law and essence of Christianity has helped me obtain a clarity of thought I had not reached before.

Les Stobbe, president of Here's Life Publishers, whose personal consultations have helped me be a much better writer.

Sharon Kay, assistant in typing and research.

Cynthia Kane, a longtime friend of our family and a patient who unselfishly invited me into her inner life so that I could learn more deeply about the dying process itself and the utter faithfulness of God in our most difficult situation—dying.

Dorthea Nyberg, an author who challenged me to write about the life-support dilemma.

Dave and Neta Jackson, trusted writers and editors who gave me encouragement and excellent assistance in writing this book.

Rev. Daniel Schemmer, my dad, who not only demonstrated for me that Jesus Christ is the source of peace and all comfort through his living, but also through his dying.

Jesus Christ, who has given me peace and solace in my own sufferings and difficult times of life; plus He has extended that same peace and comfort through me to many of the patients to whom I otherwise would have had nothing to offer. Without His working in me and through me, I honestly could not have written this book. Without Him, I too would have to ask the question: "Why go on suffering when a shot or a poison drink could save me further misery?"

CONTENTS

As a physician-surgeon and a practicing Christian, Dr. Schemmer brings light and truth to a critical problem facing medicine and theology today. Standing by the absolutes by which he lives, he recognizes the complexity of modern medicine's capacity to keep "a corpse alive" indefinitely, and the rising costs of medical care (emotionally and financially). Yet he balances his belief that every person is made in the image of the Creator and in relationship with Him with issues of the quality of life.

Dr. Schemmer understands the "slippery slope" which led Germany, between 1921 and 1944, to liquidate anyone not considered "Aryan" enough or considered handicapped in any way.

Through it all runs Dr. Schemmer's personal faith, that "for the Christian, dying is a part of one's witness to the world of God's presence and resource that goes beyond the dying process."

I'd recommend this book for practicing physicians, nurses, medical students, seminary students, clergy and physician workshops and seminars, and ethicists. Any thinking person concerned with the modern dilemma of medical support systems for the "living dead" and society's need for cost-accounting and pain relief will find this book helpful in examining the issues involved.

John Monroe Vayhinger, Ph.D.
Executive Director,
Colorado Interfaith Counseling Center,
Colorado Springs, Colorado

I am a physician, and during my 25 years of medical practice, I have helped hundreds of people recover from potentially fatal diseases and accidents to live many additional, happy years. But all of us must die sometime, so it has also been my experience to help many people go through the process of dying as peacefully as possible.

I have been particularly close at these times because I am a surgeon, there when people face the most serious medical crises such as cancer, auto accidents, and biosystem failure.

It has not been my practice, when I get called to see a patient, to go to the operating room, scrub, do my art, and disappear. Whenever possible, I stay in touch with my patients until they recover or die. Many times I take care of patients throughout a terminal illness as their primary doctor; often I am their only physician.

These patients require hundreds of hours of care beyond strict medical and surgical treatment. Some suffer terribly, not only physically but emotionally. At times the agony seems unbearable and these patients beg for relief. I do everything I can.

Sometimes, however, I have to admit that I am already doing everything possible to relieve the pain, but I assure them that I hear their cry, and I am trying to understand their horrible suffering. At those times I promise to be available to them as a friend and fellow human being. "Whenever the pain gets to be too much," I say, "call me, and I will come and hold your hand and go through the especially difficult times with you."

Strangely enough, that recognition of their agony frequently brings a sense of peace and acceptance. Somebody knows and understands. Someone is with them.

But something has been happening in recent years. Even though we haven't yet conquered cancer or reversed the process of dying for many diseases and accidents, our technology has made it possible—after a grim fashion—to defy death. We can hook the body up to one machine after another to replace its failing systems and force what remains to continue on.

Initially these "miracles" were invented to relieve a failed biosystem while it recuperated or, in more recent years, until it was replaced by a transplanted organ. All this was done with the hope that the person would one day return to a semblance of normal life. But those same machines can be connected to a dying person in such a way as to prolong the suffering of death indefinitely, forcing the person to remain in agony when their entire body and spirit longs to be released.

Because of their incapacity, these modern specters cannot participate in the life of this world, but their spirit and conscious mind is being prevented from passing into the next. Whether or not there were ever ghosts in the past, we have most certainly created the equivalent in the present.

Similarly, these same machines can be connected to the body of a dead person in order to keep it functioning indefinitely, in some cases until useful organs can be removed for transplant, in others until a court gives permission—sometimes years later—to "pull the plug." In this situation we have an animated body without a spirit or mind, or what is known in voodoo superstition as a zombie.

During my second year of medical school I worked in a geriatric hospital; later in my practice, for eight years, I was part-time medical director of a nursing home overseeing 200 people. I saw the bitter effects of people's diseases and the process of dying. Many people were embarrassed at their lack of control over their bodies. I've helped clean up patients' stools when they lost control. Whew, stool everywhere!—on the bed, patient, floor, and walls. And the terrible smell on both of us lasted for hours.

Other patients could hardly tolerate it when a nurse or daughter had to actually help them urinate, take a bath, or change their clothes. A number were deformed, paralyzed, blind, or deaf, unable to communicate simple desires or needs. Different ones knew that sometimes they said stupid, uncaring, even abusive words. Many cried and worried about the same things day after day without any sense of being repetitive. And depression over their failing health with its limitations, inabilities, and pain plagued the rest of them.

It is cruel to artificially prolong this condition beyond the time when God would take a person. But in all too many instances our "miracle machines" do just that.

I am not antitechnology. I perfect my skills with the latest laser scalpel for use in surgery and will use any other device that truly helps people. But there has been another even more frightening by-product of our enshrinement of technology. Driven by the mandate to do "everything possible" to prolong life, and drunk with the notion that we can, in fact, hold death at bay, many people are embracing the idea that the very time of death is no longer God's to determine but ours to choose.

Our grandiosity is reflecting backwards: euthanasia is being suggested with new vigor as the way to escape the pain of dying and the seeming uselessness in old age. Doctors are being proposed as the only reliable executioners. As with the abortion issue, "quality of life" questions are being introduced to determine *who* is worthy of living.

I sympathize with the life-support dilemma. The fact that such undesirable solutions are being put forward reflects the reality of deeper problems. There are several hard questions that must be faced:

- Is it wrong to want to die when you're old or in pain?
- Why wait for a natural death?
- Should we cling to life at all costs?
- Can any meaning be found in suffering?

As a Christian community, we simply must become conversant about the life-support dilemma and its ramifications, and work to solve the problems on a moral basis, or we'll lose in the legal arena like we did on abortion. The dilemma will not wait. Even today we need practical answers to questions such as these:

- Should I or a loved one go on a life-support system?
- Who will pull the plug and when?
- When is a person actually dead?
- What about taking organs for transplant?
- What is natural death?

I believe that we can discover helpful answers to these questions, answers that are informed by God's Word, the compassion of Jesus, and our Christian conscience. Therefore, I invite you to join me in the rest of this book as we consider the *life-support dilemma* from the following perspectives: the development of modern medical technologies; the legal aspects of current cases; what it means to be a person; what I, a doctor, would want for myself; and how to work with families needing answers to the hard questions concerning a loved one—a parent, spouse, or child.

Throughout the coming pages we will seek Christian, moral answers and ways to be healers and helpers in unbearably painful situations, rather than executioners.

Kenneth E. Schemmer, M.D.
Brea, California

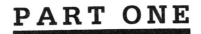

PART ONE

The Life-Support Dilemma

CHAPTER ONE

A Chilling Proposal

As a physician, I've faced many situations where the agony of my patients was so great that I longed for the Lord to take them. Sometimes I've even prayed He would do just that. And I'm sure that many of these suffering people have said with the Apostle Paul, "For to me . . . to die is gain. . . . I desire to depart and be with Christ" (Phil. 1:21, 23).

I remember Roger.[1] He was a 55-year-old man who had a cancer of the right upper lung which had grown through the ribs and into the nerves going into his right hand. He had constant, severe bone pain and nerve pain running down his arm into his hand. There was no position in which he could hold his arm or hand that would relieve the pain even a little. He could not lie down at night because lying made the pain worse and breathing very difficult. I gave him a mixture of pain medications, including morphine by the quart, to take at home.

One day his wife brought Roger into the office. He looked like walking death itself! He had not slept for almost a week. The pain was at its worst. They wanted more pain medicine, which I willingly provided. I told him that I could see he was in a great deal of pain and knew his agony. I held his hand and pledged my availability to go through the pain with him and his wife. He left the office that day with a new smile, the kind of smile one gets when he's found a new friend, a person who actually understands and cares.

But I never considered playing God and ending his life by my own hand. During 11 years of medical and surgical training and 15 years of medical practice, my entire focus has been on showing mercy to my patients by helping them fight their diseases and find relief from pain. It was a very single-minded art that I learned, reinforced by the Hippocratic Oath that has served medicine so well since 400 B.C. In affirming the Hippocratic Oath, I promised that "I will give no deadly medicine to anyone if asked, nor suggest any such counsel; furthermore, I will not give to a woman an instrument to produce abortion."

Certainly the recent advent of legalized abortion has brought a change in this ethic for part of society, but that change is often rationalized by not considering the fetus to be a human being. Some moral forecasters have warned that sanctioning abortion will certainly lead to other forms of legalized death. But most doctors consider that to be alarmist talk and would continue to fancy themselves as healers and helpers.

Doctors as Killers

Recently, I came across a proposal for "The Humane and Dignified Death Act," a piece of legislation currently being proposed by the Hemlock Society. The Hemlock Society has always advocated euthanasia, but there is a new twist to this proposal. It reads as follows:

The Hemlock Society announces the publication of the Humane and Dignified Death Act which will permit a physician to end the life of a dying patient upon the competent request of the patient. This is known as active euthanasia, as distinct from passive euthanasia, which allows a hopelessly ill person to die without prolongation on life-support equipment.

The reason for the Humane and Dignified Death Act is that there are some individuals whose suffering at the end-stage of life becomes so great that they wish to bring about their own death. The Hemlock Society states that this could not easily be accomplished, and there are many botched attempts at suicide in these circumstances. Furthermore, any person who helps with death commits a felony.

After five years of research and policy-making in this field, the Hemlock Society has concluded that the best answer to this problem is physician aid-in-dying. Under the new Act, the decision to end life will be solely between patient and doctor (with a second doctor's concurrence) and family members will be informed but not able to intervene.

There must be a legal declaration by the patient taking complete legal and moral responsibility for the decision.

The Hemlock Society does not expect all physicians to welcome this Act, but it knows that some will. Helping to die with dignity has become part of good medicine today, and those physicians who believe this deserve immunity from court action against them.

The question arises more than ever before of how the incompetent patient, perhaps suffering from Alzheimer's Disease, may have euthanasia.[2]

When I first read this proposal, I felt as if I was being torn apart. How can a physician be asked to be a killer? Healing and killing are diametrically opposed. Destroying defeats restoring. I tried to imagine what this would mean if I were the patient. How could I know whether my doctor was coming to me as a healer or a killer? Of course, the proposal says that the doctor would only be a killer at the request of the patient, but if my doctor were emotionally prepared to be either executioner or healer, I would be concerned that his or her *inclinations* might influence actions sometimes when I didn't want them to.

Bleak Implications

If such a law were enacted, how long would it be before the demand for "full services" from hospitals pressured all doctors to become killers regardless of their personal convictions? And how long would it be until court cases expanded the law's application so that doctors could be sued for costing the state or the family extra expense by not ending someone's life as requested?

Note a few of the implications that are already hinted at in the proposal:

- "Family members will be informed but not able to intervene."
- "Those physicians who believe [in practicing euthanasia] deserve immunity from court action against them."
- "The question arises . . . how the incompetent patient . . . may have euthanasia."

The prospects are chilling: even the family wouldn't be able to stop the euthanasia; the executioner could not be prosecuted; and next on the agenda is the search for a way to dispose of those who don't deserve life because of their impaired mental state. Of course, this point is euphemistically phrased to sound like these people are currently being *deprived* of euthanasia.

Nazi Parallels

Does this kind of proposal remind you of Nazi Germany? It should. There are several disturbing parallels. Robert Jay Lifton, in his book *The Nazi Doctors*,[3] makes the following observations about the Nazis' practice of genocide:

1. All nonbattlefield German killings were medical, that is, carried out by or under the supervision of medical doctors. This lies at the heart of the proposed Humane and Dignified Death Act.

2. Medical materialism lent itself directly to "purification

projects" that killed in the name of healing. Materialism focuses on the technological and the biological. In America the
unwanted, unborn person is the impurity, the disease. By getting rid of the impurity, the state and the mother's control
over her own body is "healed." In Germany, when science
included such a purification project in the name of healing the
state, professionals moved to the farthest shore of evil, such as
Auschwitz and similar exterminating camps.

*3. The claims in favor of euthanasia in Germany were that
it was an act of compassion.* But the root words of compassion
are from the Latin, *com* (meaning together) and *pati* (meaning
to suffer). Thus the word compassion basically means to suffer
with another person. We suffer together rather than to put
another human being out of his suffering by killing him. So-
called "mercy killing" may benefit the killer and serve his or
her ends more than the patient's, but that does not justify
calling it a merciful or compassionate sentence.

Killing portrayed as compassion also occurred in the names
of such organizations as "Rhelm's Committee for Scientific
Approach to Severe Illness Due to Heredity and Constitution,"
which was responsible for eliminating unwanted children.
Transportation for the patients to killing centers was carried
out by the "Charitable Transport Company for the Sick." And
the "Charitable Foundation for Institutional Care" was in
charge of collecting the cost of the killings from the relatives
without, however, informing them what the charges were for.

*4. Anything society could find to decrease the physician's
perception of the condemned people as human increased his
ability to kill for the state.* This point is extremely important,
because only through such a change in perception can a doctor become more of a killer than a healer. For instance, the
main justification for abortion is the claim that the fetus is not
really a human being.

*5. The Nazis based their justification for direct medical kill-
ing on the simple concept of "life unworthy of life."* Whether
we say the person is suffering too much, costs society too
much, is incompetent, doesn't have enough life left to profit

from his or her good organs, or is undesirable for some other reason, these are all reasons used to declare someone's "life unworthy of life" and, therefore, liable for termination.

6. *Killing in the name of healing.* Nazi rhetoric included justification of sterilization for people who had genetic diseases that "dilute the genetic pool" as though this were a healing service rendered to humanity.

Actually, the concept of killing in the name of healing recounts how the whole abortion issue began. I remember a number of young women brought for therapeutic abortions to the university hospital where I interned. It was claimed that these women would have grave psychological problems if they did not have therapeutic abortions. It was hard to prove this claim, but if two psychiatrists verified the diagnosis and then a gynecologist performed the abortions, they were permitted.

One case I particularly recall was an older teenager who came to my ward for postoperative recovery. For days after the therapeutic abortion she cried bitterly: "I killed my baby!" Yet the concept of a therapeutic procedure is supposed to mean something done with the aim of healing.

7. *The Nazis' success was in translating their most murderous actions into technological problems.* What were the objectives of those favoring the practice of euthanasia? They searched for the best techniques for quick, quiet killings. And when death occurred pleasantly, technology was quickly perceived as a part of the natural order of nature. Mercy killing in any particular case was thought to be right because it seemed as common and dignified as natural death.

Potential for Enactment

But is there a chance that we could actually endorse a law such as the Humane and Dignified Death Act in the last decade of this enlightened century? Well, in Holland, family physicians already commit over 5,000 active euthanasia killings a year. The Dutch Health Council asked in January 1987 that new legal guidelines protecting physicians from prosecution be worded so that a doctor is not obliged to consult parents or guardians of a minor when the sick child asks to die and refuses to involve them.[4]

In this country, California, Arizona, and Florida show the most interest in active euthanasia laws so far. In California, for instance, a group called Americans Against Human Suffering, Inc., produced a ballot initiative which they hoped would qualify for the general election in November 1988. This initiative, which did not get on the ballot, is none other than the Humane and Dignified Death Act quoted above.

Two other groups, one called The Concern for Dying, which has a mailing list of over 350,000 people, and the Society for the Right to Die, emphasize education of doctors, legislators, patients, and their families to the rights of patients. The stated aim of Concern for the Dying highlights programs that change the way people see the issue through quarterly conferences of young lawyers and health care professionals to plant the seeds of new attitudes for years to come.

Why do these organizations grow so quickly? A.J. Levinson, executive director of Concern for the Dying, explains the impetus: "There's a growing acceptance because there's a growing segment of the population that has had a terrifying experience, themselves or a loved one losing their rights, to medical technology."[5] That is, the problems and agony of prolonging death artificially has created a reaction which insists on the right to end life artificially.

Amoral Use of Technology

The popular backlash that has led many to embrace euthanasia will continue to mount in importance *because* our society continues to use technology without laying a moral basis for its use. By default our motto is: "If we have the technology, use it." Yet we don't know when to start it, how much to use it, or when and how to stop using it.

We have come to serve our technology instead of human beings. Furthermore, technology has gotten in the way of our relationships with the very people we are supposed to serve. Every segment of society is involved in this technological problem. In medicine it becomes most acute, for no one wants an impersonal robot taking care of him or her. We all long for that "personal touch" when we are sick and hurting. In a time of sickness, whether physical or psychological or both, what every person needs most is the relationship that only another human can give. Above all, each person ultimately desires to be treated as a human being of worth and dignity.

Not long ago I cared for a man who had extensive cancer of the abdomen. The operation was not a step in curing the cancer but of relieving his intestinal obstruction that the constant use of a tube through his nose into his stomach did not solve. After the operation, Walter recovered fairly well for several days. Then he began failing. And suddenly he suffered a cardiac arrest. He was immediately resuscitated and put on a life-support system with a mechanical ventilator, medications to support his heart action and blood pressure, and constant high-tech monitoring of his physical condition. The extent of his cancer and the profound nutritional depletion it caused had weakened his vital organs too much. He required artificial life support to live.

The next morning he motioned for something to write on. His response to the life-support system was unmistakable: "Stop! I don't want it." He was quizzed by his family, and he gave the same response. Over the next few hours he played tic-tac-toe with his daughter. This showed that he was mentally alert enough to know what he wanted. We had a long discussion with Walter and his family about the certainty of his death once the life-support system was discontinued, but he remained unequivocal. We knew that the life supports were only prolonging his dying. The next morning he continued to get weaker. So we all decided to follow his wishes and removed his life-support system. Ten minutes later his heartbeat slowed, he went into coma, and the EKG displayed a flat line: no heartbeat.

I did not feel it would have been right to force Walter to stay connected to those machines. There was no chance for recovery if he had stayed on the machines, and God took him as soon as the machines released him. But to me this is far, far different than actively taking someone's life or assisting him in taking his own life. I personally believe as both a physician and a Christian that euthanasia is not the answer. It does not address the true need: It does not support patients so they can cope with their dying, for it does not help them victoriously express the dignity which, as human beings, distinguishes us from the animals.

We must bring to the final days of our lives all the experiences we have gained over the years if we want to die congruently with the way we have lived. The use of technology can help us live longer, have less difficulty in living with some of our diseases, and make life more comfortable. None of us wants to give up the advances in medical technology that we have today. And yet none of us wants to become a slave to that technology.

Schizophrenic Roles

Reading the Humane and Dignified Death Act proposed by the Hemlock Society caused me to wonder how long a doctor could switch back and forth between the role of healer and killer without loosing his equilibrium. Would the time come when he or she might lose that keen interest in the patient's best that is so necessary for a healer? Might the time come when such a doctor would suffer from moral schizophrenia and be confused about what was to be done when?

A striking example of this very point occurred in New Jersey. Wyman Garrett, M.D., was a former member of the Newark Board of Education, member of the University of Medicine and Dentistry, and at the University Hospital, who pleaded no contest to charges of gross malpractice and other improprieties, mostly involving abortions on 40 patients.[6]

The charges he pleaded no contest to included: performance of an in-office abortion beyond the permissible stage of pregnancy on a 14-year-old who died of complications; failure to recognize and treat complications during abortions, including uterine ruptures and one case in which a fetal head was not removed; and, altering medical records on some of the patients involved in the alleged malpractice cases.

His attorney tried to defend him by testifying that Dr. Garrett had suffered intense emotional "burnout" from the stress of performing 2,700 late-stage abortions in recent years. Under the stress of these legalized "mercy killings," he had lost his perspective on his role as a healer.

Dr. Garrett took the first step away from the highest moral standard by performing any abortions. The next step—performing late abortions—became sufficiently easy for him to do 2,700 of them. Finally, so used to taking human life, he broke morally and proceeded in an utterly reckless fashion. On January 30, 1987, Administrative Law Judge Sibyl Moses wrote, "The conduct of which Dr. Garrett pleaded is so egregious, so adverse to the very minority members for whom he has stood up in the past, that it cannot be countenanced in society."

Is this an isolated case? Could physicians kill some people and help others without losing their mental balance? Possibly. It happens in war—but only by considering those one kills as "the enemy." And it happened in Nazi Germany—but look at the price. If we think it can be done with impunity, watch it happen to the Royal Dutch Medical Association.

Loss of Person-oriented Care

At the very least I fear the person-oriented approach—so important for a good physician—would give way to a thoroughly technological perspective. There would be no other way for a doctor to cope. The process of concentrating on treatment rather than the person (as we have so frequently done in recent years) would dehumanize the patient enough to make the transition between healing and killing easy. But being a physician presupposes a moral connection between the doctor and patient, as so well worded in the Hippocratic Oath.

It will be a ghastly day if our lawmakers approve active euthanasia. But tremendous pressures are at work pushing our society in that direction.

What are they? And how did they begin? Those are the subjects of the next chapter.

Notes

[1] All names in this book have been changed unless *both* first and last names are given.
[2] "Goodlife, Gooddeath," in the *Chapter Reports of the Hemlock Quarterly,* Issue 22, January 1986.
[3] Robert Jay Lifton, *The Nazi Doctors* (New York: Basic Books, Inc., 1986).
[4] *The Orange County Register,* March 31, 1987.
[5] Andrew H. Malcom, "Movement Seeks to Advance Rights of Dying," *The New York Times,* December 12, 1984, p. 1.
[6] *American Medical News,* February 20, 1987, p. 4.

CHAPTER TWO

How Did We Get into This Mess?

On June 1, 1986, Marie Odette Henderson, a 34-year-old San Francisco kindergarten teacher, was admitted to Kaiser Permanente Medical Center after complaining of feeling ill. She had been pregnant for six months without complications, but the doctors discovered that she had a brain tumor. After a week of intensive diagnosis and treatment, the brain tumor produced so much pressure that it destroyed the brain stem, and her doctors declared her brain dead June 7, 1986.

At that time, Marie's physicians also determined, however, that her unborn baby girl had only a 10-percent chance of survival if they removed the baby then. But if the baby were allowed to develop to a 34-weeks gestation in her mother's womb, she would most likely survive.

Marie had been living with her boyfriend, Derrick Poole, but they were not married. So her legal next-of-kin were her parents, Otis and Edna Henderson, who, upon considering their daughter's situation, exercised their legal rights by ordering the hospital to remove her life-support system when she was declared brain-dead. However, Derrick, the baby's natural father, quickly obtained a temporary restraining order keeping Marie and her baby on the life-support system.

Therefore, the doctors laid plans for everything they could do to maintain Marie and her pregnancy until the 34-week mark unless her body began to deteriorate or the baby developed fetal distress. The hospital set up a special operating table in case an emergency cesarean section delivery became necessary.

Although Marie was brain-dead, she had a six-month-old, live, three-pound baby girl developing in her womb. For this reason she was kept in intensive care on a heart monitor, a respirator, IV fluids and nutrition, and routine nursing care. In this state of suspended animation Marie's body provided almost all of the functions necessary for her baby's survival. Since her brain was dead, however, it did not produce any of the natural hormones which were necessary to maintain the pregnancy. So the doctors administered them artificially. The baby's progress was watched by a fetal monitor and an ultrasonic machine, which displayed a picture of the baby inside the uterus.

Then a month later Derrick got the thrill of his life: "I saw the baby on the ultrasound machine, and it was a sight to behold. She opened her eyes wide like she was looking right at me. I saw her heart beating, her knees, her rib cage, her fingers, her toes, and they were all normal. It was a feeling you can't describe."

As the weeks passed, the baby's chance of survival increased to 75 percent. And so, on July 30, 1986, baby Michelle was delivered by Cesarean section, a 32-and-a-half-week, healthy preemie.[1]

This case dramatically illustrates the *life-support dilemma:* the ability of medical technology to prolong dying and/or to extend life. In some cases physicians—with the aid of life-support systems—have kept a patient's body alive for no justifiable reason for years after the brain died. But this particular case beautifully portrays the marvelous working of doctors and the best of medical technology to keep a body functioning for seven weeks for a worthwhile purpose: to save the life of the baby.

Development of the Life-Support Dilemma

As a premed student at Purdue University in the late 1950s, I worked as an orderly in a local hospital. Helping the nurses when a patient died always intrigued me. A nurse would place her stethoscope to the patient's chest and listen for a heartbeat. Hearing none she'd then listen for breath sounds. Next she placed a mirror near the mouth to look for moisture of the breath. Satisfied that the heart and lungs had stopped functioning, she declared the patient dead.

Today at the first sign of death, the nurse calls a "code blue" and then begins CPR (cardiopulmonary resuscitation). A whole team of people appear, as if out of the walls. They surround the patient, connect him up to monitors and intravenous lines, and administer medications to stimulate the heart. If no heartbeat or a very abnormal one registers on the EKG monitor, electric paddles are placed on the patient's chest and an electric current is delivered through the chest to the heart. Frequently, at that point the heart will return to a strong enough beat to sustain its own function and that of the other vital organs.

Today many patients who are seriously ill can fully recover from a heart attack. Furthermore, a number of other conditions that cause the heart or lungs to stop—conditions that would have previously signaled death—can be reversed when neither one of those two organs has failed because of its own disease.

So technology can help us bring back the functions of the vital organs of the entire body that have temporarily stopped—every organ, that is, except the cerebral cortex of the brain, that part of the brain responsible for the higher nervous activity. But even though we can't restore the function of the brain, technology can now duplicate the function of the *brain stem,* that part which automatically controls the operation of other parts of the body.

Medical technology, in actuality, has produced a mechanical brain stem.

Benefits of Technological Advancements

In most cases these advancements have been beneficial, and even the simplest tests or observations have prevented some patients from dying needlessly.

I can recall, for instance, the first time that I knew of a patient who had a seizure and swallowed his tongue. His death wasn't due to the seizure, as had been earlier suspected, but resulted from his blocked trachea (windpipe) and subsequent suffocation. Now we pull the tip of the tongue back into the mouth, and these patients live.

Another simple observation led Dr. Henry Heimlich, one of my professors at the University of Cincinnati, to develop his now-famous maneuver to remove food accidently lodged in someone's windpipe. The use of the Heimlich maneuver has saved thousands of people who would have otherwise died.

Life-support systems are not themselves the problem. For instance, one piece of life-supporting equipment familiar to most people is the cardiac pacemaker. It can be lifesaving for patients with severe heart rhythm abnormalities and provide excellent health for many years. My aunt, for instance, had a pacemaker inserted at the age of 85, and at 90 she still lives alone taking complete care of herself. The pacemaker's use could not be construed as prolonging death.

Cardiac pacemakers come in two types: temporary and permanent. The temporary pacemaker is frequently used after open-heart surgery to regulate the heart's beat, since significant abnormalities frequently occur in the early postoperative period. When the heart rhythm returns to near-normal the pacemaker is removed.

The wires that lead from the pacemaker to the heart and conduct the electrical current that stimulates the heartbeat can be inserted through a large vein that goes directly to the heart. When the time or facilities are inadequate to place the pacemaker through the vein, a needle containing the pacemaker wire is inserted directly through the chest wall into the heart muscle. Every year thousands of people who might have died prematurely enjoy years of virtually normal life with the aid of their pacemakers.

The Common Uses of Life-Support Systems

The more total life-support systems are most commonly employed when the lungs are unable to function properly. Three conditions can cause this.

1. *Failure of the brain stem* denies the lungs the necessary regulatory signals to function. But if the lungs are artificially stimulated to work, they can supply the blood with adequate oxygen, and all the other tissues of the body can function properly.

2. *Chronically diseased lungs* may fail to adequately purify and oxygenate the blood so that the brain stem dies for lack of oxygen. When this condition exists, the rest of the body also dies slowly from lack of sufficient oxygen.

3. *Acutely injured or diseased lungs* may be functioning so poorly that death would ensue. However, if the brain stem is still functioning adequately, a life-support system can temporarily take the role of the lungs until they can recover sufficiently to support the patient's life on their own. Then the artificial system can be discontinued.

The Origins of High-Tech Medicine

The stage was set for the life-support dilemma some 30 years ago with the creation of the ICU, the hospital "intensive care unit." As new technological developments became available to the average hospital, doctors and nurses had to have a special place where they could care for these critically ill patients with their new equipment and training. And they soon proved effective in improving the care and chances of recovery for seriously ill patients.

During my 25 years as a medical doctor, I have appreciated each new development that helped me monitor patients who required intensive medical treatment. As a surgical resident at the University of Cincinnati, I used early EKG heart monitors and first-generation mechanical ventilators to help people breathe whose lungs had failed because of injury or acute lung disease. I remember a number of teenagers who had been in terrible accidents dying because we couldn't support their lungs long enough for their injuries to heal. How happy I was when newer models of the respirator became available. And better respirators inspired more vigorous monitoring as well. A breakthrough in testing for oxygen, carbon dioxide, and the pH (acid-base) levels of the blood allowed us to finely tune those new respirators and save the lives of a number of patients that we would have lost before.

Other advances have given physicians the ability to salvage many more patients who are desperately ill. These developments include the arterial blood line that constantly produces a tracing on a screen showing the blood pressure; monitors inserted through the great veins of neck or chest directly into the heart measure the strength of the heartbeat, the amount of blood the heart is pumping per minute, and, in a failing heart, on which side failure occurs. With all these new technological tools, nurses also have to have specialized training to use them correctly.

In this way, ICUs continuously siphon in more high-diagnostic modalities and therapeutic interventions of machines and monitors, more specialized doctors and nurses, and more patients who might profit from these specialized high-tech units. The result? An ever-increasing growth of higher costs to the medical delivery system.

But another result is the application of these technologies to chronically ill and dying patients causing their existence to be prolonged. In this way the life-support dilemma has become an everyday occurrence.

"All-Out" Expectations

Initially ICUs were not designed to prolong life unnaturally, but to help people recover from life-threatening illnesses or injuries which would otherwise end a normal life prematurely. Several important tenets of medical technology, however, emerged almost unnoticed.

- Each patient admitted to the hospital began to receive a high-tech workup and treatment.
- The ICU became the measure of excellence in medical care with the rest of the hospital a step down from there.
- When a patient was in ICU, he or she received all the facilities and professional attention the hospital could provide.

For those who recovered, medical science triumphed and the medical staff felt satisfied. And for those who didn't, well, at least "everything possible" had been done for them. Doing "everything possible" for a patient became the universal expectation, measured in technological terms.

Many times, however, I recall wondering what I had accomplished by treating these dying patients with our high-tech gadgets. Frequently, those patients lay in bed without ever responding to anything.

One particular teenage girl reminded me of one of my daughters. So when I would finish Ruth's medical care, I often stood and looked at her. Questions flooded my mind: "Who is this teenager? Does she enjoy school? What are her favorite subjects? Does she love volleyball like my daughter does? Does she hate spinach as much as my son does? Does she enjoy getting up early in the morning when her father arises and pulling a joke on him before he goes to work like my daughter does?"

Sometimes the questions came every day. Her family would often fill me in on the answers, but Ruth never did. And after a while my questions stopped, for only a body lay in that bed, an empty body without a person to use it.

I thought back to those first years of premed at Purdue. This same girl would have been pronounced dead the day she arrived at the hospital because we had no machines to substitute for her brain stem. But for Ruth? We were *capable* of keeping her body functioning after her brain stopped, and so we did . . . for nine long weeks.

Each time this scenario happens, many of us in the medical profession long for a way to tell who is about to die and shouldn't be resuscitated, and who might profit from our high-tech care.

Why did this life-support dilemma begin? Charting some of the historical developments that led to the current dilemma helps describe how it evolved, but it does not explain why we haven't always been able to use those developments for the patient's good. What's been the problem?

Moral Considerations Are Made Secondary

With each new step in life-sustaining technology, the fascinating mystery of death began to be unveiled before our very eyes for the first time in human history, revealing the possibility of pushing back that final moment further and further. But our moral development did not keep pace with our technological advances.

As each area of the unknown became known, physicians grew continually more interested in better methods for monitoring the patient. With more precise monitoring came more exact diagnosis. We were able to state with increasing accuracy what specifically caused a patient's death. And with that knowledge, there was the chance to attempt a corrective with the next patient.

Upon hearing of new technological advances in basic research, many physicians took problems from the patient to the lab. For instance, when I was a surgical resident at the University of Cincinnati, I spent a lot of time in transplantation research. My professor would define a problem that we saw in the patient undergoing a kidney transplant. We then went to the lab and designed a research protocol to investigate it, and then performed experiments. We figured out the problem and decided what could be done for the patient. Finally, under very controlled conditions, we changed the treatment plan according to what we had learned in the lab and proceeded with the patient's care. Frequently, this resulted in significant improvement of therapy. But in most medical circles there has been little rigorous moral consideration of the wisdom of various procedures.

A major example of how medical possibilities have outdistanced moral considerations occurred on March 27, 1986, when Baby M was born as a result of human science and two couples. Mary Beth Whitehead, a 29-year-old married mother of two children, agreed, for $10,000, to be artificially inseminated with the sperm of William Stern so that Mr. Stern and his wife, a pediatrician whose medical condition would worsen if she became pregnant, could have a baby. However, after the pregnancy Mrs. Whitehead decided that she did not want to give up her baby girl.

What began as a technological triumph became a moral nightmare. Should surrogate motherhood be allowed? And if so, how do we protect the mothers, fathers, and babies of such a technological union?

Public Demand for an All-Out, High-Tech Approach

Research groups grew up all over the country. At surgical meetings they reported their findings and encouraged incorporating these findings into daily practice. High-tech measures became more and more necessary to provide services that were consistent with the best care available. When lawsuits challenged a doctor's choices, even the courts judged the defending physician according to the latest developments in technology: "Did he do everything possible?" Medical facilities had to have state-of-the-art equipment in order to attract or keep physicians or draw patients.

Technology, therefore, set the pace for medical care. Medical students were taught the latest in scientific technology with less emphasis on their relationship to the patient as a person. Physicians were judged not so much on the basis of their "bedside" manner as their skillful use of technology in the diagnosis and monitoring of patients. It became prudent to utilize the technological advances earlier in the workup of patients rather than to take a few days to make the diagnosis by daily examinations.

Grandiose Physicians See Death as a Personal Defeat

Many physicians are so absorbed with treatments and technological possibilities that they wage a very personal battle against human mortality, and the death of a patient emerges as a personal defeat. As long as any sign of life lingers, even if only produced by a machine, they persist in continuing everything that has been started. When death triumphs these doctors suffer great guilt for "losing" a patient, sometimes ignoring the fact that they were trying to prevent that patient's human destiny.

But something worse transpires: when death proves imminent and inevitable, these doctors are into so much denial, that they sometimes have trouble relating to a dying patient.

The Christian physician knows his or her finiteness and inability to prevent death or provide the perfect treatment in every case. Therefore, when he makes mistakes—as we all do—he can confess his plight to God and receive forgiveness. And he can remain with those dying patients, pointing them to the greater hope of life with Christ.

Physicians who are not reconciled to the ultimate human destiny of death may push further than indicated with some treatments in order to take another crack at defeating the disease or mortality itself. Or the physician may be so personally preoccupied with fighting the disease or the dying process that he or she cannot respond to the emotional and spiritual needs of the patient. Unfortunately, this often happens when the patient needs the doctor's personal attention the most.

Two of my colleagues are cases in point. Dr. Reed fought with every machine, drug, and operation possible to keep an elderly woman alive—including major surgery three days before she died—despite her repeated instructions to the contrary. Dr. Adams was so emotionally involved staving off death in one of her dying patients that she was unable to hear or respond to his needs. For weeks before his death, he asked to discuss his pain medications and stop the physical therapy that produced a lot of pain, since he was dying anyway. But Dr. Adams' denial of mortality was so strong that she couldn't change anything for her patient.

The Cost of Excessive Technology

The development of the life-support dilemma occurred out of a desire to help return sick and infirmed people to normal health. There was no real thought of prolonging the dying stage. Yet this has been one of the results. And it should not be surprising, since humans don't have full control or power over life. In addition, there have been other high prices to pay.

First, the patient-doctor relationship has suffered. For example, a very common operation today involves the removal of a diseased gallbladder which has stones in it. When a patient's symptoms indicate gallstones, we first obtain an ultrasound examination of the gallbladder. This technology may be used before the patient actually sees his or her physician and certainly prior to visiting the surgeon.

This approach saves a lot of time in the doctor's office; however, it also reduces the time available for the doctor to spend with his or her patients. Likewise for the nurse. And technology certainly slashes the time spent with patients in the ICUs where patient care predominately centers around the monitors and various aspects of the life-support systems.

As medical communities have increasingly lost contact with patients, the relationship of the doctor to the patient has suffered. The very emphasis on technology has caused the *focus of attention* to shift to the technically definable aspects of the patient rather than the patient as person. With constant production of more high-tech equipment and upgrades of current instruments, the effect of all this technology has resulted in the patient getting lost in the shuffle. For example, when a particular machine causes problems and it seemes it should not be used anymore, a new model replaces it. We don't stop using machines; we just switch to better ones.

Christian psychiatrist Paul Tournier understood this problem. In his book *To Resist or To Surrender?* he says:

> Reduced to the elements of science and technique, medicine is in danger of losing its human quality, of becoming dangerously impersonal. . . . Neither science nor technique can give physicians an adequate or whole view of the human person.

Many of a patient's ills can only be understood and the burden of their disease relieved by caring, compassionate human beings, especially those of the health care team. Where this is not the case, patients fear that they will get stuck on a life-support system without meaningful personal contact. That's what denies them their sense of personal worth and dignity, not necessarily the machine itself.

Some Advances Create New Problems

Part of the life-support dilemma arises from man's inability to completely control the consequences of his creativity. At the outset of a new discovery we believe our invention will have only positive effects, but that is not always the case.

For instance, medical science thought that the development of antibiotics would provide the key to curing infection and many diseases. I remember Dr. William Altemier, my professor at the University of Cincinnati, describing how in the early 1940s, 80,000 units of penicillin would cure pneumonia. But by the 1960s we sometimes needed to use 20 million units— 50 times the earlier amount—to fight a severe infection. By then a number of bacteria began causing infections in patients who were already being treated with antibiotics, and so new synthetic ones were made that would destroy these new bacteria as well. Every few years since then new and lethal strains of bacteria have developed, and we must create ever more powerful antibiotics.

What was thought to be the answer to a problem turned out to be the beginning of new problems. In addition, some of these powerful antibiotics create serious side effects that can result in death or handicap in some patients.

The effectiveness of organ transplantation has been greatly advanced by the drug cyclosporine which reduces the body's tendency to reject foreign tissue. But cyclosporine causes toxic liver and kidney complications. In fact these very toxic side effects create considerable confusion in determining the onset of kidney and liver rejection, for at this point no clinical signs can accurately distinguish cyclosporine-induced toxicity from rejection.

Limited Resources and Death Sentences

The limited resources of medical technology push the doctor into another dilemma. Artificial kidneys are a case in point. Even if the artificial kidney functions well and patients improve, who qualifies to use one when the supply lags behind demand? And with the transplantation of organs, should one person get five or six successive kidneys—despite the tremendously short supply—when several other potential recipients haven't received their first one? Who decides this and how does he or she make that decision?

Hearts, lungs, and pancreases are in even shorter supply. By what standard will these decisions be made?

- Will it be the patient with most potential for a long, productive life from whom society will benefit?
- Will it be the person who will cost the least to cure?
- Will it be the rich who can afford it?
- Will it revolve around the quality of life, thereby excluding the elderly and feebleminded?
- Will it be the person most likely to recover?

The cost of organ transplantation continues to rise so that the value of the whole transplantation program comes into question. Should we be spending so much money on so few people when so many die of common diseases? When the kidney dialysis program started it maintained the lives of about 10,000 people with chronic renal disease. Now more than 73,000 patients receive dialysis at a cost of over $2 billion a year. And by the early 1990s the cost of dialysis could be $600,000 for each patient.

The government estimates the cost of a heart transplant in excess of $150,000 for the first year of survival and $250,000 for a liver transplant. With the estimated need at 15,000 hearts and 8,500 livers, our country could easily spend over $4 billion for one year's medical bills for these 23,500 patients. (The one-year survival rate for heart transplants is approximately 80 percent; for livers, about 65 percent.)

As the success of these transplantation programs increases, there will be more types of organs transplanted—for instance, transplanting heart and lungs together in patients with advanced pulmonary vascular disease who have damage to both the heart and the lungs, and pancreas and kidney together in diabetic patients with terminal kidney failure.

But the problem of limited resources and high cost worsens when we consider that many of those patients have other chronic illnesses which could end their lives early or add a tremendous cost to their overall care.

A Life for a Life

One of the most exciting areas in neurosurgery focuses on the CNS (central nervous system). Today's experimental investigations may permit future treatment of various disorders, such as Parkinson's and Alzheimer's diseases, and correction of traumatic and ischemic injuries of the CNS by the transplantation of fetal pituitary tissue into adults. Initial experiments have been successful in obtaining virtually normal pituitary function.[2]

But, if this becomes a common procedure, where is that fetal pituitary tissue likely to come from? Probably aborted fetuses—a very high price indeed.

Dr. Herbert J. Buchsbaum, professor of obstetrics and gynecology at the University of Pittsburg College of Medicine tells us that intrauterine evaluation can be performed by anatomic, biochemical, and genetic assessment of the fetus *in utero*. Refinements in sonographic techniques allow examination of fetal anatomic structures as small as the lip and external genitalia. The diagnosis of fetal heart defects has been expanded and can detect abnormal blood flow through the heart valves. With these techniques the major cardiovascular malformations and malfunctions can be diagnosed while the baby is still in the womb.[3]

How do we combine such dedicated research work with the tremendous drive by our society for legalized abortion? At every point of technological advancement in this field there will certainly be those who will use that technology against the fetus declaring it a "life unworthy of life" in order to justify their own desires. For along the way to diagnosing malformations so they can be corrected and thus offering a baby a new lease on life, those babies with minor imperfections could be rejected by disinterested parents. It is possible to believe that some people might abort an unborn baby only because it is the wrong sex.

As these and other medical technologies advance, the life-support dilemma will continue. Today physicians are beginning to be able, through the advances of technology, to say with a high degree of certainty whether a person is living or dead. So far, we cannot predict accurately enough to tell if the patient will recover or whether we are only prolonging death by connecting him or her to a life-support system. We cannot wait, however, until that day to address the moral issues. In the meantime our task revolves around ethical and moral considerations about human life and death and the way we relate to human suffering.

Notes

[1] John Everson, "Fetus of Single, Brain-dead Woman Poses New Legal, Ethical Issues," in *American Medical News,* August 1986.
[2] *The Bulletin of the American College of Surgeons,* January 1987.
[3] Herbert J. Buchsbaum, *American College of Surgeons Bulletin,* January 1987, p. 23.

CHAPTER THREE

What is Death?

Paul E. Brophy had worked for a number of years as an emergency fire fighter in the Boston area. On several occasions people who were overcome by fire and smoke required resuscitation at the scene. These patients often needed life-support systems while their lungs recovered, but some never recovered and were dependent upon the machines indefinitely. As a result of this, Paul had discussed with his family the possibility that he might sometime be so sick as to require a life-support system. He made it clear he did not wish to be another Karen Quinlan.[1]

On March 22, 1983, at age 45, Paul Brophy complained of a headache and then fell unconscious in bed. After being taken to the hospital he regained consciousness. The doctor diagnosed the rupture of an aneurysm of a cerebral blood vessel. His surgeon explained the delicate problem to him including the necessity of operating on the leaking vessel to prevent another bleed from killing him. He also told Paul about the risks of such an operation including the possibility of permanent brain damage or even death.

Before the operation on his brain, Paul told one of his daughters, "If I can't sit up to kiss one of my beautiful daughters, I may as well be six feet under." After the operation Paul never woke up; he remained in a coma, without moving, breathing through a hole in his windpipe. One eye remained closed while the other wandered aimlessly. His left hand was clenched so tightly that the fingernails broke the skin. He was completely dependent on others for all of his care. Because of his comatose condition Paul required a nasogastric tube (a tube going through his nose down into his stomach) to receive fluids and nutrition.

Paul continued in a permanent loss of consciousness. However, five months later, in August 1983, Mrs. Brophy and her family requested that a "do not resuscitate" (DNR) order be placed on her husband's chart. Their request was followed. But by December 1983, nine months after the operation, the medical staff asked Mrs. Brophy for permission to arrange for her husband to undergo surgical placement of a tube through the abdominal wall directly into the stomach (gastrostomy) for feeding purposes, which was performed without incident.

Several months later Mrs. Brophy—a nurse herself—asked the doctor to remove the gastrostomy tube and let her husband die. The hospital said no: "The removal of the gastrostomy tube would guarantee that a patient who was medically stable would starve to death. We felt this was unethical."

In February 1985, therefore, Mrs. Brophy asked the Probate Court of Norfolk County, Massachusetts, to issue a declaratory judgment that the gastrostomy tube should be withdrawn from her husband. After an extensive trial that included testimony by several physicians and ethicists who held that it was not ethically permissible to allow patients like Paul to die, the court permanently enjoined the staff from removing or clamping the gastrostomy tube. Furthermore, the court permanently enjoined Mrs. Brophy from authorizing any medical facility to remove or clamp her husband's gastrostomy tube.

The Probate Court found that, although Brophy himself had on several occasions expressed opposition to being kept alive artificially if his condition ever became hopeless, the state's interest in preserving his life outweighed any personal preferences. Brophy, the court found, was not terminally ill or dying, and so, because his condition was in effect "curable," the state insisted that his life be saved.

However, in September 1986, three and a half years after Paul's brain hemorrhage, Mrs. Brophy won the right to have his feeding tube disconnected when the Supreme Judicial Court of Massachusetts reversed the decision of the probate judge and ruled that the tube could be disconnected. Paul Brophy's case established that a hopeless patient whose wishes are known may have all treatment, including feeding, stopped.[2]

When one reads a story like this, it is easy to sympathize with the Brophy family and the trauma they experienced, not only over the loss of Paul but the struggle to do what they felt was right and best under the circumstances. And yet questions persist: Was there a chance that he might someday have awakened in his right mind? Was there any reason to hope that some future technological breakthrough could have revived him? Was he a sacred living soul, or was the real Paul dead and gone with only his body being sustained artificially?

To attempt to answer these questions, it may be helpful to understand the current definition of death and thereby why there is pressure to change it.

The Current Definition of Death

In 1968, an ad hoc committee of the Harvard Medical School gave a clinical definition of death that required the entire central nervous system (CNS) to be irreversibly functionless. This is sometimes called whole brain death. Its criteria rest on four important principles:

1. There must be irreversible structural damage to the CNS. (Machines can now determine this.)
2. Nothing can be depressing the brain stem's function such as alcohol and barbiturates, muscle relaxants, hypothermia, or gross metabolic imbalance.
3. Brain stem reflexes—corneal, pupillary, gag, and oculovestibular—must be absent.

4. There must be no respiratory effort during a satisfactory trial period.

If any of these criteria cannot be fulfilled, a confirmatory test to show the absence of cerebral blood flow is mandatory. But under these conditions, death is uncontested.

Demands for Revision

However, in a recent article in *The Western Journal of Medicine*, A. Craig Eddy, M.D. and Charles L. Rice, M.D. point out that victims of profound and irreversible brain damage survive longer today because of improved critical care. They therefore contend that the old definition is not helpful. They explain:

> Brain death inevitably follows brain stem death, and this death is a process, not an event. It has now become clear that spinal reflexes, auditory-evoked brain stem potentials, and electroencephalographic activity can persist after CNS death. The persistence of these neurologic functions does not alter the inevitability of death, but it often complicates the decision to terminate support.
>
> To continue artificial support following brain death deprives a patient of a dignified death and needlessly prolongs the anguish of relatives . . . exhausts precious health care resources . . . and that for successful transplantation, brain death must be established before organ deterioration precludes harvesting. Last, a clear definition of brain death is important for legal reasons.[3]

Should we heed this call for change? If so, where should the line be drawn?

The major problem in redefining death is not only technological but moral. The crux of the matter is the question of what technological and scientific data mean in moral terms. *It helps to recall that science is a descriptive inquiry and has nothing to do with the purpose or meaning of the data.*

As the issue is debated, we must be very careful that we do not change the definition of death to the detriment of any person or group of vulnerable people such as the retarded, the elderly, or the senile. And as Christians, we need to be sure we do not redefine it in any way that contradicts Scripture. We must also balance our thinking between the use of technology and relating to people as persons, not treating them as machines.

Therefore, the ultimate question of what death is can be enlightened by exploring what makes us uniquely human.

The Brain and Its Function

As long as the brain functions to any significant degree, no question exists as to whether the patient is a person whom we are morally obligated to protect and care for.

A person's kidneys may stop functioning, and he may require the support of an artificial kidney; his heart and lungs may give out and he may require a machine in assistance or replacement. Yet until the brain has failed, we know for certain that the patient is alive and human.

The focus of authentically human life lies in the function of the brain because that is what sets humans completely apart from all the rest of God's creation. Vegetable life, of course, has no brain at all, and animal life, even in its highest forms, lacks self-consciousness and the capacity to reason.

Only human beings are set above the animal world by a God-given spirit with the capacity of self-consciousness, free will, and the ability to commune with God. While there is no set of specific cells that can be called the spirit, I believe that it is the combined, higher-level operation of the brain—sometimes thought of as one's personality—that constitutes what we can comprehend as the human spirit. Therefore, a live human brain might be called the seat of the human spirit, while its operation *is* that spirit in temporal expression.

The importance of brain function is so central that the whole body serves the brain; the brain does not serve the body.

Oh, to be sure, the brain integrates bodily functions and coordinates body movements, but that is not the brain serving the body; it is the brain *directing* the body.

The most highly developed and mature cells in the body are located in the thin layer of gray matter on the surface of the cerebral hemispheres, folded into ridges (gyri) with about two-thirds buried in the depths of the fissures. This cerebral cortex of the brain is the seat of reasoning and reality, value decisions and creativity. It is responsible for general movement, visceral functions, perception, behavioral reactions, and for the association and integration of these functions—everything we associate with personality. When we understand this, we can see why the cortex so greatly sets human beings apart from all the rest of creation.

These are the cells that require the rest of the body to deliver and maintain—on a minute-by-minute basis—the proper nutrients (glucose) and circulation (oxygen) for its function. When the rest of the body reduces its care for the brain, the brain's function immediately decreases. If the body's support is interrupted, the brain begins to die very quickly. In fact, if the steady delivery of glucose and oxygen is interrupted for about ten minutes, the person will lose all cerebral function and consciousness . . . *forever.*

Levels of Brain Death

The brain dies in increments. When glucose and/or oxygen are denied, the first part of the brain to go is the cerebral cortex—that is, the outer part responsible for the highest functions—then the midbrain, and finally the brain stem. We used to think this happened as one event so that the brain seemed to be a single unit. However, with the latest diagnostic equipment, we have been able to chart the dying process and know the sequence.

As has been mentioned previously, *whole brain death* means the irreversible cessation of all brain activity. This was the situation of the patients declared dead by the nurse whom I assisted as a premed student at Purdue. It is the easiest condition to determine. The whole nervous system dies with no signs of life whatsoever as defined by the four criteria mentioned previously. This includes brain stem death resulting in the cessation of the heart and lungs. All neurologists recognize the characteristics of whole brain death.

Death of the Cerebral Cortex

Problems only arise in determining the point of death when an electroencephalogram (EEG)—the machine that can detect electronic activity in the brain—reveals that the brain waves of the neocortex (that part of the brain that distinguishes human beings from animals) are flat and nonexistent, but the brain stem is still functioning and stimulating the heart and lungs to continue operation. Is a patient in this condition still a person with all the moral rights afforded to a human being simply because his or her heart continues beating? And how much neocortical EEG activity indicates that the person remains alive enough to be himself or herself? This latter question arises sometimes because there can be a little flicker of activity called "residual neocortical function" without it indicating any hope for a return to consciousness.

Such cases are often referred to as a *persistent vegetative state*. However, the President's Commission on Foregoing Life Sustaining Treatment has recommended use of the term *permanent loss of consciousness*. In this condition, brain scans and subsequent autopsies show that the actual brain tissue has been dead for some time.

According to an American Medical Association estimate, on any given day in the United States there are an estimated 10,000 patients with a permanent loss of consciousness who are maintained by tubal feedings.

In my opinion, if neocortical death can be established, there is no justification for sustaining the rest of the body artificially. A person in this condition is utterly gone. There is no chance of coming back.

Midbrain Death or "Locked-In" Syndrome

The moral dilemma deepens when we consider the patient whose midbrain dies—say, if a cerebral arterial aneurysm ruptures or a stroke occurs. This condition usually presents itself as though the neocortex has died, since midbrain death prevents the cortex from communicating with the rest of the body, as all its signals must go through the midbrain.

James Brennan experienced this "locked-in" syndrome when, on May 28, 1986, he suffered a stroke while on the way to the Philippines for a vacation. The doctors in the Japanese hospital to which he was taken when his plane landed in Tokyo did not recognize the condition and assumed he was in a true permanent loss of consciousness, a coma.

However, ten weeks later when he was returned to San Francisco's General Hospital, neurologist Dr. Dan Lowenstein recognized Brennan's condition when he leaned over and asked him: "Can you close your eyes?" Brennan blinked, and Lowenstein said, "Welcome back to America." Tears filled Brennan's eyes.[4]

Brain scans showed massive cell death in Brennan's midbrain. However, it was at a point just below where the visual and auditory nerves diverge. Had the damage been a centimeter higher, he would be comatose, possibly with eyes that roved randomly, but focused on nothing. As it is, he is truly alive and aware and now able to communicate in rudimentary Morse code by blinking his eyes. This is an extremely rare condition. But understanding its distinctions helps us grasp the differences between *human* life and the death of what's truly human. It also demonstrates the ways doctors can now determine those distinctions.

Brain Stem Death

Presently, even when the neocortex and the midbrain units die (which almost always happen together), the patient remains medically and legally alive if the brain stem still functions.

Moreover, because physicians so frequently use life-support systems to arrest the natural dying process before the legal whole brain death occurs, we have more people with a permanent loss of consciousness than we used to have. Our problem lies in the distinction of when the dying process of the brain can be stopped so that the true *person* survives, and when, if stopped, no *person* will be there anyway.

Furthermore, as we have pointed out earlier, machines can substitute for the functions of the brain stem and stimulate the body to continue operating whether or not the higher brain is alive. Therefore, it is my earnest contention that a live brain stem does not in itself constitute a living soul and it should not be artificially preserved if the higher brain is dead.

The Absence of a Neocortex

Anencephalic infants present a unique moral problem but one which gives us a deeper insight into the life-support dilemma. Anencephalic infants are born without most or all of their cerebral hemispheres (the *absence of* rather than the death of the cerebral cortex, as discussed above). Yet, these babies are not totally brain-absent since they usually have a brain stem, and, therefore, they cannot be declared brain-dead under current laws. In this regard, it may be helpful to point out the reason for the use of the whole brain death idea in the beginning. Dr. Michael R. Harrison of the Hastings Center reported:

> The whole brain definition of death was adopted to protect the comatose patient whose injured brain might conceivably recover function. Obviously, this precaution need not and should not apply to an anencephalic who never had and can never have the physical structure necessary for higher brain activity or cognitive function. Failure of the brain to develop is clearly different from injury to a functioning brain, and was not considered when the "brain-death" definition was formulated.[5]

Each year about 3,000 babies are born with anencephaly. Because of the near total lack of the brain 60 percent of them die within 24 hours of birth, and only 5 percent live more than seven days. None of them have any feelings, not even to pain.

While anencephalic infants die very quickly despite life supports, their situation brings up the question of whether to use their hearts, livers, and kidneys as transplants for children who are otherwise normal except for one vital organ which is failing.

The current estimation puts the annual need in the United States at between 400 and 500 infant hearts and kidneys, and up to 1,000 infant livers. Therefore, the nearly 3,000 anencephalic infants born each year could supply the needed organs for all the children who need these transplants to survive. Several people have suggested that the anencephalic babies could be put on life supports when the diagnosis is secured to maintain their bodies until the transplantation of the organs was accomplished—the procedure that best prevents any deterioration to the organs. But then, under the current definition, the cause of death would have to be listed as "the removal of vital organs."

A Canadian couple with an anencephalic daughter was the first to choose to "wrest something good from their tragedy." The heart and lung of their baby, Gabrielle, now beat and breathe in a baby named Paul, who would not be alive except for their gift. The procedure they followed technically stayed within the letter of the law. When Gabrielle could no longer breathe on her own, she was attached to a respirator and flown from Toronto to Loma Linda University Medical Center in California. There the doctors took her off the respirator and declared her dead before removing her organs.

This successful transplant was performed by Dr. Leonard Bailey, the same doctor who placed the heart of a baboon into a 12-day-old baby, extending life for an additional 21 days.

But *if* anencephalic infants are human spirits in God's eyes, then there is no excuse for using them as a means to achieve an end, no matter how compelling that end might seem. If one exception is made (i.e., taking organs from a human with a living soul), the list of candidates could get very long, including the retarded and the mentally senile. Therefore, we must resist the pressure to change the *law* until there is a clear resolution of the *moral* question of what constitutes human life.

At this point in our technological understanding, we know that the human being can exist without (or with a replacement for) every part or organ of the body except one and still have the essence of what distinguishes humans from the animals. That one component is the neocortex.

Therefore, I must draw the line between human life and death at the cerebral cortex. When it is alive, I believe we are morally obligated to defend that person's life to the fullest. When it dies, the human person expires too. When the neocortex dies, it can never be revived and neither can the person.

Yes, we do need to redefine death so that it reflects our best spiritual and medical understanding of when a person remains in the body and when that person has departed. To use our modern technology in life-support situations demands that we bring our moral understandings up to date. But that's not the whole story. There are some *very* critical qualifications that must be attached to any new definition.

Determining Death

The progress of diagnostic technology to redefine death in terms that accurately denote the functioning of a human being has begun to increase in the past few years. In the later part of the 1960s, various medical centers began to report patients on life-support systems who had complete absence of all brain-wave activity (as determined by EEG) whose readings were identical to the readings of patients not on life supports who had recently died, having no heartbeat or respiratory activity of the lungs. In other words, their brains appeared to be equally dead.

During those years I can remember several young, healthy

adults who had suffered severe head trauma from accidents. When the EEG showed complete brain-wave inactivity for at least 24 hours, clinical death was pronounced, but the life-support system was continued until kidney transplantation could be accomplished. However, some people could not accept the complete absence of brain function as the measure of human death because they felt that as long as any organ functioned, the person was not dead, and they held out hope for recovery.

This led to a dual definition of death: (1) the cessation of breathing and heartbeat—the traditional determination, and (2) the irreversible cessation of all brain activity including the brain stem, even if the body could be kept functioning artificially by high-tech machines.

Efforts to Upgrade Diagnostic Ability

In an attempt to bring our diagnostic technology up to the state of the art that had been reached in life-support systems, a lot of research has been done on brain functioning and its relationship to the dying process and death itself. These have included measuring cerebral blood flow by using xenon-enhanced CT scanning of the brain, brain imaging with magnetic resonance, chemical brain biopsy, cerebral spinal fluid (CSF) analysis of large intracellular molecules which have leaked from damaged brain cells, and the measurement of enzyme peaks resulting from the whole brain which has been deprived of adequate blood and oxygen from various causes of brain damage.

The concern initially was not so much the detection of whole brain death as it was defining and then diagnosing the death of the cerebral cortex alone.

Currently, the legal definition of death requires a whole brain death standard (technologically determined) that duplicates the traditional cessation of heart and lung activity. In other words, we still see a person as a full-fledged human being even when we know that he or she has no ability or potential to fulfill any of the requirements of what it means to be a human being.

A Recent Breakthrough

Part of the dilemma we face in patients with a permanent loss of consciousness occurs precisely because of that unconsciousness. Is the patient's cortex dead (so there is no hope of ever recovering)? Could they be unconscious but recoverable? Or could they actually be conscious but unable to communicate by usual ways as we saw in the locked-in syndrome?

Until quite recently, these distinctions could not be made with certainty. But now Dr. Fred Plum, professor in the Department of Neurology at the New York Hospital-Cornell Medical Center, and his associates have developed the technology needed to differentiate those patients who have cerebral cortical brain death from those who do not.

Using positron emission tomographic (PET) measurements of regional cerebral blood flow and glucose metabolic rate, they discovered there is no metabolic overlap between vegetative patients and either normal or locked-in persons. They also found that even patients with marked cerebral atrophy could not be confused on the CT scan with those in the vegetative state (complete cortical death).[6]

What this means is that *for the first time* since we began hooking people up to machines that replace their vital organs, we can now determine whether we are keeping *a person* alive or just *a body* functioning.

For Christians and all who are concerned with our moral responsibility to protect the sanctity of life, this is a most welcome breakthrough. It may provide us with our first truly ethical release from one aspect of the life-support dilemma.

Plum's group found that even though some vegetative-state patients exhibit a lot of organized motion as a reaction to different stimuli,[7] it does not mean that the cerebral cortex is functioning, even at an undetectable level. All it means is that the spinal cord and the brain stem are active.

As to the locked-in syndrome, they assert that even though "the locked-in state superficially resembles the vegetative state . . . the clinical distinction is almost always straightforward and based on the ability of locked-in patients to communicate using coded eye movements." They further stress the need to show great compassion and sensitivity when caring for locked-in persons because, "despite their profound motor loss, these persons feel, think, and experience anguish in close to a normal way."[8]

Practical Use

Positron emission tomographic (PET) scans currently are done in only a few centers across America and are moderately costly. Therefore, this technology is not commonly available. But the primary contribution of Plum's work was to *confirm* the detectable distinctions between unconscious patients, locked-in patients, and patients with a dead cerebral cortex.

Fortunately, there is a cheaper and widely available test that can be used, now that these distinctions have been proven to exist. It is the pulsed Doppler ultrasound (PDU) measurements of the carotid artery blood flow, and it can be done in any hospital in America and is accurate by itself.

Recently published research states that "no patient had the characteristic brain death waveform without being clinically brain dead, and no patient who had cerebral perfusion by angiography had a brain death waveform. This indicates a high level of specificity for the characteristic waveform seen with brain death."[9] This is to say that when the characteristic brain death waveform is present, even though the brain stem may be functioning and sustaining heart and lung action, the cortex is reliably dead. Furthermore, "measurement of carotid arterial blood velocity with pulsed Doppler ultrasound is a repeatable, noninvasive, portable test useful for confirmation of brain death."[10]

What does all this actually mean in the care of dying patients? It represents a landmark discovery: the actual clinical point of death of the human being can now be identified technologically with certainty. We no longer need to worry about pulling the plug too soon. When a patient has all the clinical evidence of permanent loss of consciousness over a period of time, we can now obtain a PDU test and a confident determination of brain death.

If there is any question, PET studies of regional cerebral blood flow and glucose metabolism can be pursued and proof can be obtained whether the patient's cortex is definitely dead or not.

This sets a new standard upon which to define human death, and legal rulings will have to be established to employ it. But for the Christian, it provides the most tangible way to cope with the life-support dilemma without giving into the pressure of euthanasists.

Notes

[1] Karen Ann Quinlan was a 21-year-old comatose woman on a respirator. In 1976 the New Jersey Supreme Court issued a landmark decision granting her family's request for her to be disconnected. The court reasoned that she had a legal right to refuse treatment and allowed her father, as the next of kin, to render his best judgment as to what she would want. Unexpectedly, she survived in a coma off the respirator until June 1985.

[2] Philip R. Reilly, J.D., M.D., "Physician Defends Feeding Man in Coma," *American Medical News,* February 14, 1986. Also, Mark Rust, *American Medical News,* September 26, 1987, p. 23.

[3] A. Craig Eddy, M.D., and Charles L. Rice, M.D., "Brain Death, *The Western Journal of Medicine,* June 1987, pp. 738–739.

[4] Lisa M. Kreiger, "Spirit Stays in 'Locked-in' Body," *San Franciscu Examiner* as reprinted in the *Chicago Tribune,* August 10, 1986, Sec. 3, p. 4.

[5] Michael R. Harrison, M.D., in *American Medical News,* April 17, 1987.

[6] Fred Plum, M.D.; David E. Levy, M.D.; John J. Skditis, Ph.D.; David A. Rottenberg, M.D.; Jens O. Jarden, M.D.; Stephen C. Strother, Ph.D.; Vijay Dhawan, Ph.D.; James Z. Ginos, Ph.D.; Mark J. Tramo, M.D.; Alan C. Evans, Ph.D, "Differences in Cerebral Blood Flow and Glucose Utilization in Vegetative Versus Locked-in Patients," *Annals Of Neurology,* Vol. 22, No. 6, December 1987, pp. 673–682.

[7] Plum's article identified the organized motion as follows: "Nearly all regain sleep-wake cycles; many display the facial appearance of interest; and

some even show emotional fluctuations with occasional infant-like tearing or smiling in response to non-verbal stimuli. Although none follow moving objects consistently, some occasionally move the eyes slowly toward visual stimuli. Others blink inconsistently to visual threat, startle or close the eyes in response to sudden noises, or demonstrate reflex groping or sucking."

[8] Ibid.

[9] Peter A. Ahmann, M.D.; Timothy A. Carrigan, M.S.A.E.; David Carlton, M.D.; Brad Wyly, M.D.; and James F. Schwartz, M.D., "Characteristic Common Carotid Arterial Velocity Patterns Measured with Pulsed Doppler Ultrasound," *The Journal of Pediatrics,* May 1987, pp. 723–728.

[10] Ibid.

CHAPTER FOUR

What Is Life?

We have confused our understanding of life by applying the word to different things. Does "human life" continue if only the physical body is functioning after the neocortex of the brain has died? Some claim that it does and, therefore, must be protected. But how much of the body must function in order to qualify as that which we consider sacred? All the rest of it? Half of it? Would it be considered a human life if even a small portion of it were still alive? The human fingernail, for instance, continues to "live" and even grow for a short time after the rest of the body has completely stopped and been buried. Certainly that is not the life we consider human and sacred.

We must have a more satisfactory definition of life.

One task that confronts us today arises out of the public's lack of understanding of the meaning of "technologically sustained life." But equally important is the task of sharpening our understanding of what it means to be fully human.

The Deficiency of a Technological Approach to Life

Technologically, man is considered a machine. In some medical circles the biological structure and function of the patient receives preeminence because only they can be measured and calculated.

But if we try to understand what constitutes life from an exclusively technological perspective, then we end up looking at a human life in the same way we look at a machine. The basic concern for a machine focuses on its continual functioning. As long as the machine does its job, then we continue using it. If it breaks down, repair it or replace the failing part, but keep it going! If not repairable, then its life ends. This approach with people, however, ignores the patient as person and relates to him or her as a "robot" with no opportunity for being fully human. Just like a robot which can be analyzed and have a failing part replaced, so the human body can be managed with spare parts. And practically every part of our bodies can be substituted for, and with a replacement part the body can continue functioning.

Yet a person amounts to so much more than a machine. Even the greatest robot of the future will never fully replace or duplicate the human being. For the human being has a meaning to his or her existence far beyond the robot. The human has purpose in and of himself or herself which does not depend on any other part of the creation, only the Creator. And every facet of human life has meaning for the whole of the human existence: birth, life, and death.

Another deficiency in the technological approach arises when a machine can't be repaired: we usually discard it. But if we relate to humans that way, we soon encounter a vast number of people who, because of retardation or elderly dementia, can't be "repaired"; yet we cannot dispose of them. Currently, approximately 2.5 million people in the United States suffer with dementia. Chronic progressive diseases such as Alzheimer's disease cause dementia in many people.

Whenever we look at the human patient as only a robot— the best of the machines—we lose perspective on what we are ourselves. The more we treat the patient as robot, the more robotic we become. If we are not careful, technology becomes the standard of life, and finally we come to serve technology as our master. Then man is truly lost in the shuffle, and the caretaker and the patient are dehumanized. Finally, we all become human robots, upgraded, repaired, or replaced accordingly to utterly practical criteria.

Our caretaking, therefore, must be person-centered: humans giving of self to other humans. Technology can and should be used but only as an aid. If we use technology without a valid purpose, we will use it for its own sake.

What Is a Human?

Possibly one of the most helpful things in comprehending what human life really means can be discovered by considering the value God placed on His creation of humans in the first place. David speaks of this in Psalm 8.

O Lord, our Lord, how majestic is Your name in all the earth!

You have set Your glory above the heavens. From the lips of children and infants You have ordained praise because of Your enemies, to silence the foe and the avenger.

When I consider Your heavens, the work of Your fingers, the moon and the stars, which You have set in place, what is man that You are mindful of him, the son of man that You care for him? You made him a little lower than the heavenly beings and crowned him with glory and honor.

You made him ruler over the works of Your hands; You put everything under his feet; all flocks and herds, and the beasts of the field, the birds of the air, and the fish of the sea, all that swim the paths of the seas.

O Lord, our Lord, how majestic is Your name in all the earth!

Our Days Are Numbered

Some people approach life fatalistically, believing that God has set the day and the hour of their death and nothing can end their life sooner or extend it longer. Throughout history this confidence has given Christian martyrs the courage to remain faithful to the very end.

Unfortunately, it has caused others to shun even the most basic medical treatment, thinking that until their "time has come," they stay invincible.

But what does the Bible say about this question as it relates to the use of life-support systems and the possibility of extending life? Here are some relevant Scriptures:

- Man's days are determined; You have decreed the number of his months and have set limits he cannot exceed (Job 14:5).
- The length of our days is seventy years—or eighty, if we have the strength (Ps. 90:10).
- Show me, O Lord, my life's end and the number of my days (Ps. 39:4).
- Who of you by worrying can add a single hour to his life? (Matt. 6:27)
- For He will command His angels concerning you to guard you in all your ways; they will lift you up in their hands, so that you will not strike your foot against a stone (Ps. 91:11-12).

This final Scripture was the one that Satan quoted to tempt Jesus to prove Himself by leaping off the peak of the temple. However, Brother Andrew, "God's Smuggler," who has taken great risks to spread the Gospel, notes that "the only paths with God's protection are the paths of God's will." He says that Jesus wisely refused to "tempt" God's protection by doing something foolish.[1]

The remarkable fact that God has extended our free will so far as to let us determine our spiritual destiny suggests that we have similar choices concerning our physical life and death. God is not duty bound to insulate us from the consequences of our actions or the actions of others. By various means, life can end prematurely, meaning before God would have preferred it to end.

But what about extending life? "Man's days are determined," Job declares. Certainly *worry* can't extend them as Jesus pointed out in Matthew, but Psalm 90:10 suggests that people's strength can vary their life expectancy by ten years or so, and God personally extended Hezekiah's days by 15 years by curing his fatal disease (Isa. 38:5). So there do seem to be some biblical possibilities for variation. Can good health care be one of the things that adds "strength"? Can an operation, medication, or even a machine overcome an otherwise fatal illness?

Was the "determination" of Hezekiah's days with or without the added 15 years? Certainly God knew ahead of time that Hezekiah would pray and ask for the extension and that He would grant it. But before that God said, "You are going to die; you will not recover" (Isa. 38:1). And certainly Hezekiah would have died apart from the extension.

This paradox between our actions and God's sovereignty presents us with something that we may never comprehend fully in this life. However, we must still chart a course that is both as humble and faithful as it can be.

A Lifeline and Its Dates with Death

We may gain some perspective on this mystery by looking at the lifeline of 93-year-old Mrs. Jennings. Last year I responded to the emergency room call on her behalf because she was suffering an intestinal blockage. The intestine became gangrenous, and she would have died without an immediate operation. A couple of months after the operation she had a massive stroke and finally did die.

Mrs. Jennings' Lifeline			
BIRTH	MATURITY	DYING	
+————————————+————————————+————+—+			
Dates with Death: A		B	C D

Date A, "premature" and avoided by medical intervention.
This occurred when Mrs. Jennings was about 33 years old and
had an ectopic pregnancy. At that time she was bleeding to
death, but an operation saved her life and she enjoyed the full
return of her health, allowing her to raise her two sons. At the
time of the ectopic pregnancy she had been in excellent
health, so bleeding to death would have cut short the length of
her expected life by 45 years.

Date B, avoided by medical intervention and careful living.
Mrs. Jennings required an appendectomy, from which she recovered. However, she was also at the end of her "normal life
expectancy" and had entered the "dying" phase of her life
characterized by the general degeneration of her whole body.
From this she could not recover, but she could delay its final
effects with medication, diet, and extra rest. After the operation she was alert and took care of herself. She lived at home.
Her children enjoyed spending time with her, took her shopping, and provided help with the housework.

Date C, barely avoided by medical intervention. Though the
medical treatment alleviated the immediate crisis of the gangrenous intestine, the trauma of the operation resulted in
another crisis in itself, making the whole procedure fairly ineffective. It did not bring about a new lease on life. Mrs. Jennings did not return to her home but was confined to bed.
Many people require a life-support system at this point. It is
here that we usually speak of "prolonging life." Often it prolongs death instead. It can be called the time of artificial life.
No one knew how long she might live or to what degree she
might recover.

Date D, unavoidable even with medical intervention. Her
stroke was treated because the extent of it could not be established with certainty until some time had elapsed. Soon there
was a second stroke, and despite the use of a life-support
system she died within a week. From the time of the second
stroke she could not communicate and did not respond to
anything. So the use of life support added nothing to her life.
It did keep her blood rich in oxygen and nutrients, but these

were not helpful to her.

Preparation for Departure

Before the advent of modern medicine, if people avoided a premature death (Date A), they simply died at Date B. Therefore, we can see that advanced surgery, antibiotics, and some of the life-support systems have helped give many people a significantly new lease on life in which they resumed many of their normal daily activities.

Most people during this time have the energy and time to get their affairs in order, make a will or change an existing one, do a number of things that they would like to do before they die, such as mend faulty relationships with family and friends and review their life to bring it all together into a more meaningful picture. Dr. C. Everett Koop, surgeon general of the United States, says:

> Right now, I am 70 years old and in excellent health. If my kidneys shut down tomorrow, let's say, after a severe infection, I don't know how long I would want to be on dialysis. It would be foolish and a waste of resources for me to have a kidney transplant at my age. I would probably opt to clean up my affairs, say goodbye to my family, and drift out in uremia.[2]

This final period of life can be very fruitful both for the dying person and the family. One can even "teach" others what has been learned throughout life that may help make others' lives better. Sometimes the reins of a business or a project can be effectively transferred to a family member or partner so that the patient can have the satisfaction of knowing that his or her work will be carried on by a future generation. But more important for the patient is the strengthening of his or her relationship to God.

Eventually, however, the patient begins the final phase of dying from which there will be little if any reprieve. Even if a life-support system is employed to sustain the signs of physical life, the personality of the patient usually drifts. As life wanes more and more, the patient withdraws and finally becomes uncommunicative and isolated. Sometimes this results from the exertion necessary to communicate; sometimes it involves the desire to not be a burden on others.

Tragically, loved ones frequently withdraw from a suffering person in this time of great need. The wife who warmly kissed her husband on the mouth, shifts to a quick kiss on the cheek, then a peck on the forehead, and finally only a squeeze of the hand. Friends who visited daily, start missing, and finally fail to show up at all.

To a degree this is understandable; we may be serving our own inclination to start separating from the person we know will soon be gone. But isn't this a time when we should forestall meeting our own needs for the sake of easing someone else's suffering? How else can we expect a friend to walk through the valley of death with courage if we leave him or her alone?

The giving of oneself to another in this dying process can bring a closeness to the very nature and sacredness of life that may never be found at any other time. In my own experience, these intimate times have provided rare and exquisite glimpses into the meaning of life that have given me a storehouse of treasures showing that God is abundantly good and loves us beyond degree. He faithfully provides compassion and comfort at such times the likes of which I have never found otherwise.

So much meaning and comfort can be found in the transition experience that to cut it short by deliberate action would make both patient and caretaker losers.

An Artificial Extension

In my opinion, the artificial phase of life consists of the prolongation of life and death at the same time. Unless the brain dies, in which case the doctor pronounces the person dead, one cannot say whether a person is alive or dead. For that person is *dying!* When a person is in this final stage, striving to revive him or her and attempting to reestablish a satisfactory level of health remains futile. We cannot stop death. (Could this be the essential message of those Scriptures that speak of our days being numbered?) In the final stage, therefore, forcing the body to function until the last tissues have failed beyond all support in no way prolongs true life.

The reverse is also true. Stopping life-support systems when their continued use offers no hope of recovery does not hasten the end of real life, because a forced existence beyond this point means only the extension of dying. Here one cannot talk about omission being any part of commission.

The major problem occurs then when the patient's condition cannot be determined to be terminal and beyond significant help. When this occurs, life support should be used until a determination can be made. At given intervals reassessments can be made, and if no progress has been accomplished, the life-support system can be withdrawn. To continue life support indefinitely without any improvement contributes nothing to the patient. (Improvement means some concrete signs of returning personality, at least some purposeful neocortical activity.)

The Bible's Definition of Life

I have suggested that human life requires a functional neocortex, for the biblical concept of the human being consists of body, mind, and soul. However, one cannot divide a living person into three separate parts, for these three aspects intertwine and function as one unit. The technological dilemma of the life-support system has shown us this in an interesting way. It shows us that the human body (biologically speaking) does not account for those unique aspects that differentiate humans from the lower animals. A person loses all his or her uniquely human qualities when the brain dies, not when the body does. The bodily functions can be replaced by machines or transplanted organs, and the patient remains a human being, provided his or her brain continues to function. But when the brain dies, the body itself—even if kept alive by machines—is not a human person anymore.

King David recognized the unity between the body, mind, and soul when he spoke in this way:

> I am always thinking of the Lord; and because He is so near, I never need to stumble or to fall. Heart, body, and soul are filled with joy. For You will not leave me among the dead; You will not allow Your beloved one to rot in the grave. You have let me experience the joys of life and the exquisite pleasures of Your own eternal presence (Ps. 16:8-9, TLB).

Life from a biblical perspective consists of much more than maintaining our biological functions or even our mental consciousness. In fact, life, in its most complete sense, is unity with God, while death is separation from God. Obedience, reconciliation, and relationship bring life. Sin, estrangement, and isolation bring death.

These alternatives began in the Garden of Eden. They recurred as the choice Moses presented to the Children of Israel at the end of his ministry: "See, I set before you today life and prosperity, death and destruction. . . . Now choose life" (Deut. 30:15, 19). And they continued as the whole objective of Christ's ministry.

The Role of the Body

Whenever the Christian considers the issues of life and death, this larger truth—that true life is found in obedience, reconciliation, and relationship—must inform any consideration of what happens to the body. Not that the fate of the body is insignificant but, on the contrary, its very presence makes us holistic beings. Consider Christ's *physical* death which signified His separation from the Father as He bore our sin in purchasing our salvation. And His *physical* resurrection demonstrated His victory over death, a cornerstone event for the

Christian faith throughout the centuries. What happens to our physical body is not the whole picture, but it stays nonetheless intrinsically tied to the ultimate meaning of life and death.

However, what about the converse? Forcing the physical body to function when the soul has departed causes a definite incompatiblity with the Bible's understanding of true life. When body, soul, and spirit hold together, the Bible speaks holistically—a living human being, made in the image of God. But when death divides them, the body stays behind as nothing more than a "temple" or "house" that will soon return to dust while the *person* goes on to be with the Lord or to suffer eternal separation from God. The body, then, embraces the human being as a whole person—body, mind, soul—made in the image of God.

To Stay or Go

This larger picture of the whole person enlightened Paul as he discussed life and death in Philippians 1:20-25, 29.

> I eagerly expect and hope that I will in no way be ashamed, but will have sufficient courage so that now as always Christ will be exalted in my body, whether by life or by death. For to me, to live is Christ and to die is gain. If I am to go on living in the body, this will mean fruitful labor for me. Yet what shall I choose? I do not know! I am torn between the two: I desire to depart and be with Christ, which is better by far; but it is more necessary for you that I remain in the body. Convinced of this, I know that I will remain, and I will continue with all of you for your progress and joy in faith. . . .
>
> For it has been granted to you on behalf of Christ not only to believe on Him, but also to suffer for Him.

In this passage one can find the following principles concerning life, death, and suffering:

1. True dignity at the moment of death comes not from

avoiding suffering but in the courage to exalt Christ in spite of pain.

2. Nonetheless, *desiring* to be with the Lord is not wrong, so we should never scold old or suffering people for praying that the Lord will take them.

3. The *reason* for "remaining in the body" focuses on the work God has yet for us to complete.

4. In verse 29 and other New Testament passages, we see that suffering is a privilege (possibly even part of our work, cf. 2 Cor. 1:5; Phil. 3:10; 1 Peter 4:13) and, therefore, not in itself a justification to abandon life.

5. On the other hand, by deduction we might conclude that because of the greater desirability to "depart and be with Christ," it would be undesirable (possibly wrong?) to try and hold on to physical life on this earth at all costs.

Of course the question still remains: "When is one's work done?" Obviously, only God can answer that with certainty. But if the above perspectives are valid, they would greatly narrow the field from the euthanasists who claim it is legitimate to voluntarily end life on the one extreme and those who would try to prolong life at all costs on the other.

This broader perspective on the meaning of life is why Paul reminded us that "death has been swallowed up in victory" (1 Cor. 15:54). We do not need to fear or flee from either suffering or death. Because of Christ's victory over death, we know that the picture is bigger than what happens to the body; therefore, death has lost its sting.

Surgeon General Koop spoke to this point very personally:

All such talk [about the end of life] has different connotations for the Christian than for the non-Christian. My wife knows I do not believe in being ushered out of this life with a lethal injection. I want to hang around long enough to be sure my family is taken care of. But after that, I don't want my life prolonged in great discomfort when it is fruitless.

I don't look forward to the manner in which I am going to die. But I do not fear death. Indeed, the way in which we face death is a matter of faith. For the Christian, it is not the end.[3]

Notes

[1] Brother Andrew, *A Time for Heroes,* (Ann Arbor, Michigan: Vine Books, 1988), Chapter 10.
[2] C. Everett Koop, M.D., "The End Is Not the End," *Christianity Today,* March 6, 1987, p. 18.
[3] Ibid.

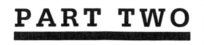

PART TWO

*In Search of
Positive
Alternatives*

CHAPTER FIVE

Bedside Decisions

Some of the absolutes by which I try to live and practice medicine include my belief in the existence of God, the reliability of His Word, the value of each person, the importance of human relationships over technology, and my unwillingness to participate in euthanasia. My absolutes do not, however, extend to *always* or *never* using life-support systems, or *always* or *never* being willing to unplug them.

Though my deepest convictions provide ethical boundaries in the most extreme situations, I still face the need to participate in some very hard decisions. The kind of decisions you may have to make if you or someone you love faces the potential of having certain operations or going on some form of a life-support system. For the elderly the challenge can involve the very hard decision of whether artificial feeding should be started or stopped. For instance, consider this case:

The phone message from the patient's daughter is ominous. "Mrs. F. has eaten nothing all weekend. What should we do?" A 70-year-old woman with severe dementia, Mrs. F. rarely speaks, is confined to a wheelchair, and requires diapers because of incontinence. She has been kept out of a nursing home by the efforts of a devoted family and daily attendance at a geriatric day-care center. During the past year, her social interactions have decreased, and her food intake has become increasingly erratic. First, she stopped feeding herself; now, even though she is fed by hand, her intake continues to decline. Once, she required admission to the hospital for dehydration. During the past week, she has been clamping her mouth shut, pushing food away with her hand, or spitting out food. Over the weekend, even coaxing with her favorite foods was unsuccessful. The question that those who care for her have dreaded must now be faced: If hand feedings continue to fail, should a feeding tube be inserted?[1]

Perhaps the best way for me to suggest a helpful decision-making process in caring for terminally-ill patients would be to explain how I proceed when confronted with the life-support dilemma. The point of the process lies in trying to make the morally best decision for the patient involved. Remember, however, I operate in the context of a patient-physician relationship. That means that *I* am a part of the process, and I must not go against my own highest moral judgment.

Part of my moral judgment must center on what is best for the patient. My moral basis honors the personhood of the patient. Therefore, I tend to see every patient as a whole person and not just a body, not just a bundle of nerves or emotions, but a person made in the image of the Creator and in relationship with God.

The checklist I use for instituting life support was developed largely by Dr. Max Harry Well of Chicago. It focuses on three principles, sometimes called the three Rs, by asking what is: Rational, Redeeming, and Respectful?

Is It Rational?

On a biological basis, does the proposed treatment make sense? That means, will it really help the patient get well or ease the pain of the sickness? Do we know what will likely be accomplished by using it? Or should it actually be considered experimental with unproven value?

If the treatment or procedure does not have a very strong chance of helping the patient, or if it probably will cause the patient additional harm, it is irrational. Similarly, if I am not sure of the patient's diagnosis or a number of unknowns about the illness or the effects of the treatment remain, it may be irrational.

Is the treatment experimental? If the scientific basis for using it has not been explained or if no solid research has been done on it, then its use must be considered experimental. If the patient cannot give adequate, informed consent for such experimental treatment or procedure, its use stays irrational, and I am morally obliged not to use it.

Many times the family will request an experimental treatment for a terminally ill patient because they don't know what else to do and feel *something* must be done. We have already seen some of the problems that have come from a go-for-broke mentality. Doctors as well as frightened family members can fall into this trap, sometimes out of fear of being sued if they do not do everything possible. But good intentions don't make a treatment rational or morally acceptable. Doing something out of ignorance just to be doing it certainly serves only ourselves and it may cause great harm and suffering for the patient.

Is It Redeeming?

Modern medical warfare can be brutal, and so we must ask whether any specific procedure will cause the patient more pain and suffering than benefit. Will the patient biologically improve enough to offset the complications which the treatment may produce? And very importantly, will the procedure significantly reverse previously lost functions?

Countless times I've seen patients given treatments for days, weeks, or months, with great hope that the patient will recover enough to go home and enjoy a "good life." Yet, these same patients often have already lost mental functions that would make this impossible even if they survived.

The farthest end of the question of whether or not a procedure will produce a redeeming result occurs when only the hope of survival dictates its use without considering its known risks. Too often doctors keep on reaching into their bag of tricks until all hope disappears. Unfortunately some of these tricks hurt and hurt badly.

The doctor does not suffer from what he or she does to patients. So it's easy to proceed with treatments even when the probability of actually helping the patient remains quite small. But if we consider the pain and suffering that the patient must endure, we would not start most of those marginal treatments.

We cannot let the end justify the means.

Is It Respectful?

What we do with and for a patient must reflect what that person wants. For many people life on a support system would be intolerable. They would give up hope and become quite depressed. But if a patient of sound mind decides to wage an all-out war for another few days or weeks of life, that is worthy of respect too.

But all too often families and physicians, afraid of the guilt of "giving up," assume they must make a massive assault on the dying body. Interestingly, at the Christa Senior Community, a Christian retirement and nursing home in Seattle, 95 percent of the nursing home residents with an average age of 86 preferred a "no code" directive for their care, indicating that they did not want all-out CPR efforts made on them if they had a heart attack or stroke. First of all, their faith had helped them come to terms with death, but they had also witnessed many friends dependent on machines, and they didn't like what they saw. The prevailing attitude among residents was: "If you can't bring me back whole, don't bring me back."[2]

Treating Patients as People

But the crux of the problem lies in our attitude. We are to treat patients as *people* and provide them with the respect due them as human beings with the God-given right of self-determination. As far as possible (while remaining morally responsible for our own actions) this must include allowing our patients to make choices we ourselves might think unwise. In so doing we treat them as an end in themselves, not a means to our own ends. Since the dignity of the patient comes from God, we honor that dignity, actually promote it, by helping them (within the bounds of what is morally permissible) to live and die according to their own sense of God's priorities for them personally.

A Patient's Rights

The patient's right to choose between accepting life-support procedures or being allowed to die without them remains essentially a moral question, for the *legality* of such a freedom has been firmly established in law.

The courts consider the decision-making process to include:
1. Ensuring consent and protection.
2. Reasonableness and usefulness.
3. Competency of the patient to make a decision.
4. The physician's duty: tell the patient the options available.
5. Standard of treatment in the community.
6. The incompetent patient has the same rights as the competent.
7. The decision-making process must include the family and/or surrogates and adequate consultation with other medical professionals if significant confusion exists.

Through all of the technological advancement of the past 30 years a persistent echo has been heard from the patient's side: a competent patient has the right to decide to accept or reject any therapy, even lifesaving therapy. And the more that sophisticated technology lengthens the dying process, the more insistently patients demand to have a say in whether or not to go through that experience. Many patients would rather die than be dehumanized by a machine. Overwhelmed by the fear that technology will prolong their suffering, some people ask to be mercifully killed.

Distinctions from Euthanasia

Is there any difference between a conscious person rejecting life-support measures and a request for a lethal injection? Euthanasia advocates claim there isn't. Both, they say, are deliberate decisions to die. If society permits one, why not the other? Meanwhile some of the most ardent anti-euthanasia leaders—afraid of a moral "slippery slope" where one concession inevitably leads to the next and then another—have gone to the other extreme of insisting on using all of the life-support measures possible, a policy that has led to some of the tragic aberrations we've all heard about.

But there *is* an important and legitimate distinction, one we must articulate with clarity and vigor. Anytime we decide a patient actually requires a life-support system, whether the most elaborate heart/lung machine or just a simple tube for feeding, we admit that the body cannot live on its own. It is ready to die. From God's perspective, that person faces one of those legitimate dates with death. It is *not* a premature date as would be a lethal injection. That's the difference!

The late Joseph Bayly told about a godly friend of his who had endured with courage and acceptance the burden of cancer for many months. In the hospital he lay weak and dying.

His doctor had told him and his wife that he could not live longer than a week or two. One Sunday night after a beautiful final visit with his wife, alone after her departure, my friend pulled the needle that was sustaining his life from his arm, shut off the valve, rolled up the tube, and went to sleep. The next day he died.

Did he take his own life? No, I believe not. What he did was merely to remove the means by which the doctor could delay his death for a few days, prolonging the suffering of his wife, delaying his soul's flight to God.[3]

However, if the patient expects to temporarily use the life-support system because its use provides a reasonable hope of recovering his ability to live independent of it, then I would urge the patient to accept the treatment as strongly as I would encourage life-saving surgery, antibiotics, or any other remedial medical treatment.

Still, the law allows anyone to refuse any treatment, and it should. Medicine is not an exact science; we cannot predict with 100 percent certainty whether a treatment will be beneficial or not. Neither can we play God. If God allows a person to encounter a date with death, we cannot judge whether He has more work for him to accomplish or not. We may have an opinion to express, but the responsibility for the decision stays with the patient.

Again, the distinction turns on the point of whether God has allowed the date with death or the patient takes it upon himself or herself to create the date.

As for the slippery slope, we will deal with it more thoroughly in Chapter 8. Suffice it to say that we will never be able to hold our moral ground if we retreat to untenable positions.

The Danger of Deciding for Others

Several states—California, Florida, New Jersey, and Massachusetts among them—now allow a person with a permanent loss of consciousness, that is, without neocortical activity, to have his or her tubes delivering food and water to be removed to allow the body to finish dying as the mind has. But the decision-making process can get complicated, as seen in the case of Nancy Ellen Jobes.

In 1980 Nancy Ellen Jobes was married, employed as a medical technologist, and expecting her first child. But the promise of her future was abruptly halted by an auto accident. It left her with a broken pelvis and took the life of her unborn child. During surgery to remove her dead baby, an anesthetic accident curtailed the blood flow to her brain. The lack of oxygen left Jobes severely brain damaged.

Nonetheless, she survived in a nursing home in stable condition for the next seven years, requiring no life support other than a tube for food and water.

Finally her family won the approval of the New Jersey Supreme Court to have Nancy Jobes' food and hydration withdrawn.

This decision was made in spite of the testimony of Allan Ropper, M.D., and Maurice Victory, M.D. Dr. Ropper is an assistant professor of neurology at the Harvard Medical School, and Dr. Victor is the coauthor of the widely used textbook, *Principles of Neurology.* These two experts examined Nancy independently and found her to be aware of her surroundings. Ropper, for instance, claimed that she accomplished eight out of twelve simple tests, such as lifting her leg, moving her toes, sticking out her tongue, and following his finger with her eyes. He attributed her failure to complete four of the commands to fatigue and stress.

The New Jersey court, however, found them to be "biased witnesses" because they were opposed in principle to removing food and hydration and accepted instead the testimony of other doctors who examined Nancy later.

Unfortunately, 32-year-old Nancy never received the benefit of a brain scan in her diagnosis, and she died on August 7, 1987, two weeks after having her food and water cut off.[4]

Maybe Nancy's neocortex was dead by the time the other doctors examined her, or maybe her responsiveness was suppressed by the medication and disorientation of the move she underwent before the later tests (the opinion of some who disagree with the court's decision). If she had been capable of expressing her wishes, would she have wanted her life support stopped? I do not know. But this case demonstrates the serious complications that can arise when others—even family members—try to make such decisions for a patient if that patient has not explicitly expressed his or her preferences when competent.

"I Can't Go On Like This"

When patients say, "I can't go on like this," it does not necessarily mean that they want to die or even that they are rejecting life support. It could mean several things, all of which could be satisfactorily improved by the determined attentiveness of the caretakers, the patient, and his family or friends.

We must be careful in all our deliberations about the delivery or nondelivery of care to patients. We only withhold treatment when the patient is terminal, near death, and when it would prolong dying rather than living. Furthermore, we should always provide total care, including fluid and nutrition, to all living people unless they reject it after being informed of all the ramifications and all their options of treatments.

The Cost of Treatment

In his *Reader's Digest* article "Medical 'Miracles' Cost More Than Money," Dr. A.E. Miller, Jr., tells the story of his patient, Emma:

> Overweight and hypertensive, she called one day to complain of chest pain. I ordered her to the hospital.
>
> That was my mistake. While signing into the emergency room, she collapsed. Six times her heart stopped, and six times it was shocked back into rhythm.
>
> But from the time of her fall, she never showed the slightest hint of brain activity. She was kept alive for eight months by a feeding tube into her stomach. If the tube had not been inserted in the first place, she could easily have been allowed to die. Removing the tube once it was inserted, however, was another matter. . .
>
> With the excuse of "saving lives," and with a little tech-

nology, I have justified tortures worthy of the Inquisition. The relatives of these patients have been twisted to the breaking point by the wonders of modern medicine.

Protracted dying is an American epidemic. The total bill is inconceivable. For Emma, it approached $100,000.[5]

Some elderly people do not want all their estates used up by the high costs of medical measures that may provide uncertain benefits. It means a great deal to them to have something to leave to their children. How does one weigh these considerations in determining whether or not to begin or terminate life support?

Resources Are Limited

Increasingly, we must consider the cost/benefit ratio to the individual, the family, and the whole society. Medical costs continue skyrocketing while available nursing facilities and personnel for the care of the elderly continue declining. Soon our nation will be looking at radical alternatives to this situation.

The government has already started to make some of those decisions for us. Currently it costs over $25,000 per bed per year for nursing-home care, excluding any special costs, with most patients on welfare. Nursing homes are often full with waiting lists, but the government has already decided to not subsidize the construction of new nursing homes in spite of the fact that the number of people eligible for nursing homes will double in the next 20 years. To this degree a decision *has been made* that society is no longer willing to pay for protracted nursing-home care for its elderly.

We will discuss several alternatives later such as hospice care, visiting nurses, and geriatric day-care centers. Remember that the cost of prolonged intensive care is simply becoming prohibitive. Facing this fact may help us moderate our "do everything possible" mentality. Just because something can be done does not mean that we are guilty of neglect when we don't choose to do it.

Individual or Group?

As a member of the human race, each person has some definition as a human being based upon his or her membership in the whole race. To that degree, the rights for one must be possible for all. On the other hand, the human race reaches its most noble expression when it makes profound sacrifices on behalf of the individual.

An example of our capacity for corporate heroics on behalf of an individual was the rescue of little Jessica McClure from the well down which she fell in Texas in October 1987. People all over the nation—even the world—prayed and waited anxiously in front of their TV sets watching brave workers make an all-out effort to rescue this one infant. However, this great outpouring of concern ironically contrasts to our nation's lack of care for the estimated 9,750 infants who died by abortion in this country during the 58½ hours that Jessica was trapped in the well.

In this case, no conflict arose between the needs of the individual and the many, but the ability to maintain perspective is hard. A conflict of interest sometimes occurs with high-cost medical care, which reduces further our ability to make a right decision. For instance, what should be done when there are only a limited number of livers available for transplant and one wealthy person who has rejected two wants a third while another patient—maybe more compatible with the available organ—can't afford the operation?

Our only hope to transcend our tendency to polarize—to opt for what is most selfish (I want what's good for me, and let the rest of the world look out for itself) or pridefully egalitarian (we won't do for anyone what we can't do for everyone)—occurs by seeking our Creator's perspective. Only God has such infinite love for each individual that He can help us see the whole and evaluate whether we can justify a great expense in a specific case. Sometimes there may be better uses for those resources.

The Food and Water Controversy

The food and water controversy is sufficiently important that it deserves separate treatment. On one hand, the idea of providing a person with food and water seems like nothing more than normal care. And it sounds barbaric to contemplate starving a person to death. But when responsible caretakers consider withdrawing nutrition and hydration, they aren't talking about denying a hungry patient their steak and potatoes. They aren't even talking about refusing to give them bread and water.

This question only comes up when it involves pumping a nutrient paste into a patient's stomach through a tube in his nose or through an incision in his side or when receiving IV fluids through a needle in a vein.

These relatively simple procedures have saved the lives of thousands of people who temporarily could not eat or drink enough to keep their bodies healthy. But they have also been used to force-feed elderly people who did not want to eat. And they have been used to sustain excessively weak or comatose patients who could not eat. In the latter case, artificial food and hydration forms the primary life-support system required to sustain many patients with a dead neocortex but a functioning brain stem.

The Legal Decisions

In 1981, in a situation known as the Barber Case, two California physicians were at first charged with murder for withdrawing nutritional support at the request of the family of a patient who sustained an irreversible coma but had an active brain stem. But the court acquitted the doctors, reasoning that supplying nutrition and hydration by artificial means was *qualitatively* the same as supplying oxygen by a respirator: "Medical procedures to provide nutrition and hydration have their benefits and burdens which ought to be evaluated in the same manner as any other medical procedure."

The New Jersey Supreme Court then followed with the same thinking in a case in 1985 in which it did not recognize any significant distinction between artificial feeding and artificial breathing or any other form of medical treatment. The President's Commission report on the issue essentially agrees.

The basis of these opinions rests on the assertion that withholding or withdrawing artificially administered nutrition and hydration does not equal abandonment of the patient; it only *allows them to die.* The switch in therapy goes from the attitude of trying to cure a dying patient to one of providing compassion for the dying. If the patient cannot swallow and does not want artificial measures taken, he receives none. He dies without receiving food or water artificially which could prolong the dying process and possibly increase the suffering.

Not So Easily Decided

But the issue is not so easily settled. Some argue that providing food and water does not amount to a medical measure but to "basic care" that everyone deserves. True enough, but it's not the *provision* that's in question. It's the *delivery system.* A tube placed through the nose or surgically inserted in the abdomen is unquestionably a medical measure, and though less complex than a ventilator, little basis remains for making a distinction when one considers that oxygen is at least as basic as food and water.

But groups like the International Anti-Euthanasia Task Force are worried that malevolent forces will take advantage of any relaxation of the law. Mary Senander writes:

> Increasingly, in what is a clear attempt to hasten the death of medically vulnerable human patients, artificial feeding is being considered optional "medical treatment." Across the nation, court cases have undermined protections for the lives of patients who are not necessarily "old," or comatose, or even terminally ill in the usually understood sense. When an 89-year-old woman was denied food and fluids for six

days until her death at a Minneapolis hospital—even though she cried out, "water, water"—few eyebrows were raised. . . .

To intentionally withhold food or fluids from a patient with the purpose of hastening or causing death is to encourage a cruel death. Beyond the physical cruelty, it undermines a fundamental trust between members of the human family. . . .

Artificial feeding is neither extraordinary nor heroic. . . . (A respirator takes over the function of the lungs; a feeding tube does not take over the function of the stomach.)[6]

It should be noted that this last claim is not entirely accurate. A respirator only *delivers* oxygen to the lungs in the same way that a nasogastric feeding tube delivers food to the stomach. The lungs must still absorb the oxygen and excrete carbon dioxide. Both stomach and lungs must continue their vital functions. There is no real difference.

However, if someone was denied food or water when they wanted it, I consider that criminal. Even when food and water are given to a patient by tubes, most patients still want some liquids by mouth unless it makes them vomit. The mouth gets dry without some water being put into it. Virtually all non-comatose patients will ask for something by mouth often up to the last minute of life. And it should certainly be given to them.

The Physical Consequences

To healthy people, the idea of starving to death sounds grossly cruel, but to the terminally ill, feeding tubes may only prolong the process of dying, and in some cases create a lot of pain and secondary discomfort. As death approaches most patients naturally reduce their fluid intake, sometimes because other bodily systems cannot handle it. Moderate dehydration can bring relief from:
- catheterization,
- bed wetting,

- frequent vomiting,
- coughing and congestion,
- choking and drowning sensations,
- painful swelling from water retention.

Furthermore, some demented patients must be tied down and sedated to prevent them from pulling out the tubes.

On the other hand, artificial hydration can sometimes provide the following benefits, especially if an electrolyte imbalance has developed:

- increased alertness and sense of well-being,
- less restlessness and disorientation,
- less nausea,
- relief from cardiac arrhythmias.

But artificial feeding and hydration often bring a decrease in human contact with the patient. When family and friends see their loved one "all wired up," they develop the common tendency to "not touch" for fear of breaking something. In some cases, therefore, hand feeding that provides inadequate nutrition or personally giving the patient chips of ice and little sips of water—insufficient though they may be—may meet more of the patient's deepest needs than tube feeding or IVs that deliver adequate calories and fluids impersonally.

Defining Goals

All of this leads us to the need to clearly define the goals of care for each patient. Is the objective to keep a dying patient as comfortable and peaceful as possible? Or is our goal to postpone death as long as possible? When the objective is clear, then the proper balance of treatment can be better determined.

1. When the patient is alert, I believe that their will in the matter must take priority, especially if they are terminally ill.

2. When demented patients stop eating and cannot be fed by hand, the physician and family must carefully weigh the benefits and burdens of tube feeding. If the feeding problem seems temporary, artificial feeding and hydration should be unquestioned. If the patient has no irreversible life-threatening problems, then long-term feeding might be indicated. However, when a patient has irreversible life-threatening problems, it may be inhumane to burden the patient with artificial food and water just so they can die a short time later from some other much more painful cause.

3. *When a patient is comatose,* I feel the primary consideration requires an evaluation of the depth of the coma and the potential for regaining consciousness. If there is no reasonable hope for recovery, then I do not see a qualitative difference between artificially delivered food and water, and artificially delivered oxygen via a ventilator.

These few examples demonstrate some of the decisions that must be made at the bedside by the patient, family, church fellowship, and physician. But to understand these decisions better, we must look deeper in the next chapter at the ethical foundations that underlie them.

Notes

[1] "Sounding Board: Guiding the Hand that Feeds," *The New England Journal of Medicine,* Vol. 311, No. 6, August 9, 1984, p. 402.

[2] Jeff Crandall, administrator, Christa Senior Community, Seattle, Washington, in an interview with Neta Jackson, March 30, 1987.

[3] Joseph Bayly, *The Last Thing We Talk About* (Elgin, Illinois: David C. Cook Publishing Co., 1969), p. 33.

[4] *AMA News,* August 1987; Rita Marker, "State Authorized Death By Starvation," *OP-ED OPINION,* the International Anti-Euthanasia Task Force, August 7, 1987; and an interview with Rita Marker, November 25, 1987.

[5] A.E. Miller, Jr., M.D., "Medical 'Miracles' Cost More Than Money," *Reader's Digest,* December 1987 p. 103.

[6] Mary Senander, *Op-Ed/Opinion* (Stubenville, Ohio: International Anti-Euthanasia Task Force) Sept. 30, 1987.

CHAPTER SIX

Ethical Foundations

The other day I discussed a case with a nurse. The patient had cancer that required the removal of his rectum. The nurse asked why such an operation would be considered after the cancer had already spread to the patient's liver—a fatal development. I explained that many rectal cancer patients have bleeding, pain, and the constant urge to defecate for many months—sometimes for a year or more—before the cancer in the liver causes death. Therefore, only removal of the rectum prevents these problems. He responded, "I guess that's a quality-of-life question."

Quality Versus Sanctity of Life

Yes, a good physician always considers the quality of the patient's life. Yet today some people have pitted the *quality of life* against the *sanctity of life*. They claim that if the quality of a person's life does not meet some arbitrary standard, the person is unworthy of life itself. This philosophy immediately places at risk the elderly with dementia, the profoundly retarded, and possibly the severely handicapped—old and young. Depending on who makes the quality of life decision, almost every human being at one time or another could be judged as possessing a life no longer worthy of living. It is one thing to strive to improve the quality of someone's life; it is quite another matter to suggest that if that effort fails, the person should die.

The Sanctity of *Human* Life

I have used the neocortical death of a patient as the determining line between actual human life (which must be considered sacred) and that which no longer represents a human soul. Some people may say that I have introduced a quality-of-life criteria. However, the actual point of my argument lies in my belief that a dead neocortex does not just *impair* the quality of life but leaves the patient *outside* the realm of what is human life—the human soul no longer residing in the body. Such a body cannot act as a human, cannot do anything uniquely human, cannot exist on its own, and has no potential (as a baby or even a fetus does) of ever doing any human activities.[1]

Some Eastern religions hold all life as sacred, and yet the product of that view makes human life in those cultures very cheap. The Bible tells us that God created humans a little lower than the angels but clearly superior to the rest of creation (Ps. 8:5-8). According to Genesis 2:7, it was into the human body only that God breathed a living soul. We should appreciate all life as a creation of God, but only human life is sacred and must be defended.

Why must we be careful to preserve those distinctions? If we attempt to defend a human body *from which the soul has departed* as though it were a human being, we will betray the sanctity of that very distinction God placed on human life, and we will end up cheapening human life as do the Eastern religions that deny the distinction.

Futhermore, as technology develops, its bizarre feats will multiply far beyond what we experience today. If we have not observed God's distinctions, but try to defend every "living" thing with a human chromosomal pattern (e.g., a body or part of a body being artifically sustained or grown), our credibility will crumble. Our efforts will not be defensible biblically or logically. The first groups who will suffer from our defeat will be the fetuses, the elderly, the retarded, and other defenseless humans who truly deserve our protection from those who do not recognize the *true* sanctity of human life.

Before our technology could substitute machines for seriously failing organs, the physician pronounced the patient dead when his or her cerebral cortex died.[2] It has been only in recent times (and as the exclusive result of our technology) that anyone could make such a body appear to be a living human being for an extended length of time. We can understand this initial confusion because we did not know about levels of brain death. And as Michael Harrison of the Hastings Center adds, "The whole brain definition (of death) was adopted to protect the comatose patient whose injured brain might conceivably recover." But now that confusion must stop. We cannot continue thinking of a body as a human soul simply because its biological apparatus can be forced to continue performing. The Bible tells us that for the believer, to be absent from the body is to be present with the Lord (cf. 2 Cor. 5:8). We must accept this as fact.[3]

So the issue of the sanctity of life rests on the presence or absence of the soul. The dying person remains a living human being until his or her soul has, in fact, departed. As long as a patient continues as a living human being, then, despite the quality of life, he or she deserves all the rights of a healthy person.

In terms of the example of the man with cancer whose quality of life improved by the removal of his rectum (even though he later died), we must differentiate between giving *quality care* and judging whether the quality of another's life is worthy of life. In the first case, the concern focuses on the patient's best interest. What can I do that will help the patient, improve his condition, restore him to a better health, or at least help him cope with or transcend his suffering? This has been the motive of the medical profession throughout the ages.

The Quality of Whose Life?

In the second case, the quality of life question gets applied to the quality of the caretaker's life. We saw this in the examples from Nazi Germany where people were exterminated for the supposed welfare of the state. Abortion advocates claim that there should be no unwanted children. However, long waiting lists of adoptive couples demonstrate that the quality of life argument applies more to the mother (sometimes merely in terms of convenience) than to the baby.

In terms of whether to begin or continue life support, economics obviously plays a role, but sometimes this also reflects a question about the quality of someone *else's* life. I have seen families compare the cost of care for an elderly grandmother or grandfather to the financial needs of a grandchild's college education, the building of a new house, or even a long-awaited trip.

In the final analysis, the application of the quality of life principle becomes a sanctity of life question. Consider how this occurred in Nazi Germany.

Nazi Dr. Pfannmuller said, "The idea is unbearable to me that the best, the flower of our youth, must lose its life at the front in order that feebleminded and irresponsible asocial elements can have a secure existence in the asylum."[4]

Behind the quality of any human life must be the "sanctity" of that life. If quality means anything, it must have a higher standard—something that authenticates it universally, at all times and in all places on the earth. We understand that a humanistic view of humankind, which sees a human being as the highest being with no superior Being, is not good enough. For the Creator sanctifies human life. He puts upon each segment of creation its place and value. When He made us in His image, He sanctified human life, made it of utmost value and supreme worth, which forms the basis for the dignity of all humans.

Let's consider the origins of World War II. Germany declared war on the rest of the world in order to have—as they claim—a higher quality of life: the superhuman race. But in order for them to have this higher quality of life, the rest of the world had to honor the sanctity of German existence, not witholding from it anything that would hinder its progress to the supposedly higher level. So in the name of the "quality of life," the Nazis sacrificed the sanctity of life for millions of people.

In the end, Germany lost its quality of life in submission to the sanctity of life demanded by the rest of the world. Oh, what ruin they reaped.

Does it ever really pay any of us to try to increase the quality of our lives at the expense of another's? Jesus said that the attitudes, the judgments, the motives, and the actions by which we deal with others determine how others relate to us (Matt. 7:1-5).

The Value of a Standard

There must be a standard from which all care emanates, or the quality of care will vary too greatly, particularly in cases where the patient is most vulnerable to the power of others. For example, I believe that the standard of care should be centered on the sanctity of life so that as long as a person remains a living human being, that person should be treated as a whole person regardless of his or her condition. For the terminal patient, we should do everything to relieve the pain and suffering and always treat the person with the highest dignity deserving of a human being. Never should we treat patients as nonpersons by injuring them or taking their lives away because we cannot relieve their pain.

Avoidance of pain at all costs is an unobtainable standard. Actually, as we will see further in Chapter 10 on the "Psychology of Death and Dying," some very important tasks in the fulfillment of an individual person can be partially met even in his or her dying—even in the midst of pain—if we will provide a person-to-person rather than a person-to-thing relationship.

As we grapple with this search for what is right, it may be

useful to briefly consider two approaches to moral reasoning: utilitarianism and causality. These two approaches seem to form the opposite ends of a spectrum.

Utilitarianism holds that the *consequences* of a course of action form the point of greatest concern in decision-making. By extension, it claims that right decisions are those that bring the greatest good for the greatest number of people.

Causality, the principle of cause and effect, claims that there is a specific, established rule for every situation. Where we have God's explicit word on an issue, we do have such an established rule that we trust. Because of His authority, we can trust that He can see and weigh all consequences better than we can.

But on the life-support dilemma God has not spoken specifically. Furthermore we can see that neither a purely utilitarian or cause-and-effect approach embodies the whole truth. If we apply a specific, established rule to every situation, we may fail to take adequate account of the consequences. But if we consider only the consequences, we fail to develop any helpful rule of conduct.

Most of us have learned that we look to both of these perspectives whenever we must make a moral decision on a critical matter where God has not spoken directly. The judgments you may have reached about the morality of war or its conduct may be useful examples. We move toward specific rules by evaluating the consequences evidenced in the past or projected in the future for various given situations.

For the Christian, we must always measure these by other biblical commands, examples, or ideals that may relate to or parallel the issue in question.

A Spectrum of God's Will

In their book *Glimpses of Glory,* Dave and Neta Jackson suggest that every decision we make can be understood as falling on a spectrum of God's will that looks something like this:

A SPECTRUM OF GOD'S WILL
(1) Biblical Commands (2) Interpretations (3) Personal Call (4) Wisdom (5) "Tea/Coffee"

The Church's Role

◀ More authority   Less authority ▶

On the left are God's commandments, clearly stated in Scripture. To violate them is sin in all situations. Next on the spectrum might fall the rules of God which need some interpretation in their application. . . . Next on the spectrum are God's desires for us personally. Some of these vary between situations and individuals. . . . Toward the right end of the spectrum are choices between good and better in terms of what is wisest. In these choices we are becoming refined into the image of Christ, but God is working very much with the individual allowing freedom without condemnation. Finally, on the far right end are choices between "tea and coffee" in which we would be claiming a false piety to think God's will supported our choices.[5]

Most decisions in the life-support dilemma occur at point 2 on the spectrum; they require careful interpretation of God's Word. There are no commandments that clearly state: "Thou shall not extend someone's life artificially" or "Thou shall not pull anyone's plug." If the technology had existed when Moses received the Law, God might have said something explicit—this issue has that kind of importance.

But the fact that God did not issue explicit directions in this matter does not mean that He has abandoned us. By the Holy Spirit He promised to guide the church in searching out what we should do as new moral issues arise. The church is called, therefore, to an active role in discerning the mind of Christ on this matter.

It is hoped that this book will form a component of that search.

The Harmony of Right Goals

In Christ Jesus, God shows us that the essence of life comes in serving Him, and serving humanity is the way to serve Him on earth. Because God has arranged it this way, the *real* good that we do for others never opposes what God asks us to do for Him.

Our relationship with God forms the essence (the stuff or meat) of the relationship He asks us to share with others. Even our behavior, then, reflects in society what He requires in our relationship with Him. Therefore, Jesus could say:

> " 'Love the Lord your God with all your heart and with all your soul and with all your mind.' This is the first and greatest commandment. And the second is like it: 'Love your neighbor as yourself.' All the Law and the Prophets hang on these two commandments" (Matt. 22:37-40).

God has designed life so that all He does helps us to love each other in the best possible way. There is no conflict. We learn the essence of love, compassion, and comfort by receiving His love, compassion, and comfort in our daily lives.

As our Creator, God knows our very nature and what is truly good for us better than we know ourselves. And isn't this the basis of morality: love, compassion, and comfort? True morality is not just the right action, but also the motive, the desire and reason for doing something, and the attitude, manner, and feeling we give to the person we serve.

As our Creator, God can judge what is best for everyone. When we try to judge solely according to the consequences, we must balance the greatest good for the individual with the greatest good for the rest of society. And therein lies the problem. First of all, human beings have imperfect knowledge of the good and frequently great difficulty in consistently accomplishing it. Furthermore, what appears as the best course of treatment for specific patients could cost the rest of society more than it can pay to provide that same option to all patients. For example, our society may not be able to provide heart, lung, or liver transplants for everyone who needs one. How do we decide who will go without?

The Golden Rule

Immanuel Kant helps us by pointing to the principle of consistency: "So act that thy maxim can be a universal maxim."[6] To do otherwise would be to commit a deep moral inconsistency.

D. Elton Trueblood, philosopher and theologian, expands on this by saying, "Each of us does desire for himself that he be treated as an end and not a mere cog in some other machine."[7] This principle helps us treat each person—whether ourselves or others—as ends and never as mere means.

While the application of these ideas does not automatically solve our problems, their careful consideration in each case aids us in asking what we ought to do so that we can at least decide what we ought *not* do. This highlights the Hippocratic injunction to first of all do no harm.

Christ's Golden Rule—"Do to others as you would have them do to you" (Luke 6:31)—forms the basis of our relationship to others. Again Trueblood helps us see what this means as a moral basis for treating our patients:

> We must, in trying to treat our neighbor as ourselves, not merely ask what he wants, for his wants may be perverted. We must not even be satisfied with asking what we would want, in his place, for our wants may be inadequate also. We must ask what we would want for him if we were perfectly loving and if we could know all of the consequences to follow from an intended act. These, of course, are impossible conditions, but they are not, for that reason, meaningless. Much of the glory of human life lies in the practical relevance of unattainable ideals. We do not achieve them, but they provide a beneficent disturbance and they indicate a standard in the light of which we can see that what we do is wrong.[8]

In a medical situation, doctors who fear lawsuits if they don't do everything possible may assume you wish to take that approach too. Sometimes one way to seek more objective advice is to ask the physician: "What would you recommend if she were your mother?" We always need to reach for the highest ideal.

Dangerous Shoals for the Physician

But how do we deal with our inability to consistently reach these high ideals? The medical profession can only attempt to save lives and promote health. Doctors themselves develop illnesses from which they cannot recover. Unquestionably, our knowledge remains incomplete, our ability to diagnose is fallible, and our ability to give the right treatment in every case is faulty.

The Immorality of Grandiosity

Here lies a point of potential immorality: *to behave as though we can do more than we can do.* At this point integrity must continually be pursued. When we think we can do a perfect job, we approach the patient as if we are God rather than human.

When we use our medical high-tech as an attempt to eliminate our human limitations to the point that we do not face up to those limitations, we deceive ourselves and our patients. And such use of technology returns us to an immoral position.

It is this attitude that allows us to exert our opinion and will over that of the patient's. In so doing we behave immorally in a second way: depriving others of their own free will. At times patients may not want to accept what the doctor considers the best treatment for them. Nonetheless, it is our duty as physicians to respect patients as persons who have the right to chose what should be done to them. They also have the responsibility to work with the doctor to accomplish their own healing. In this sharing of respect and responsibility doctor and patient can arrive *together* at what will be done.

Care of the Incompetent

Another potential for immorality occurs at the point of care for the incompetent. Here the moral health of the medical profession shows up most visibly.

Mentally incompetent patients comprise a very vulnerable group of persons. The trend to abuse them became legal with the Supreme Court's *Roe vs. Wade* proabortion decision. Now the attention of this trend has focused on elderly incompetent people in a most blatant form with the proposals for active euthanasia. If the medical profession bows to this trend, I believe that as a profession we will lose our moral respectability.

Ethicist Paul Ramsey says, "The ethical rule of practice should be the treatment of incompetents always in the way normal patients would be treated." In a particular case, then, we must find out what the usual patient requests—the standard medical therapy or not—to help us form the basis for giving it or not giving it to the incompetent patient. However, since every patient is a unique person with something different in his total situation than others, specific facts about him or her may call for another decision.

Certainly, as we have seen, the dilemma of using life-support systems presents us with some very difficult choices. Therefore, we must proceed carefully or we will slide down the slippery slope.

Practical Conclusions

Morally, the physician's job requires rendering the best medical care possible. Then the patient may have the health he or she needs to live life as fully as possible. Part of this medical care, of course, focuses on easing pain and suffering as best we can. The best interest of the patient, however, may not be served if our primary aim in treatment concentrates on relieving *all* pain. Is it better (or simply easier) to drug someone so completely that he or she is insensible to pain—and everything else?

We serve patients best when we recognize that technologically we may not be able to relieve all of a patient's pain. Why not? Because all the perception of pain does not come solely from the physical ailment. A significant portion of any pain that seems unbearable can be addressed and lessened when the caretaker becomes involved in sharing in the patient's pain and suffering. In other words, suffering much pain in isolation can make an unbearable situation for anyone. Sharing that pain—sharing resources, compassion, and comfort—not only makes the pain bearable but often allows the patient opportunity to mature through the painful experience.

We can genuinely ease pain and suffering by entering into another's pain through the comfort and compassion of a personal relationship. How does all this translate for me in a medical setting?

- Respect the person.
- Live out compassion, comfort, servanthood.
- The patient first, me last.
- Work for the patient's good, not harm.
- I only assist God in His healing ministry.
- Where I fail, I needn't despair; God can still help, comfort, and bring meaning and value.
- Be the best person I can so I can give my best to others.
- Never take human life, destroy its potential, or possibility.
- Don't try to prevent the inevitability of death.
- The pursuit of good health does not mean grasping at immortality but the best use of what God has given us.
- All of life can contribute to our maturing.
- In pain, suffering, agony, and even death, God remains in charge of cause and effect, and works for our good.
- In any dilemma there is always another option, God's option.

Notes

[1] As seen earlier, the absence of these functions does not in itself equal the departure of the soul. In the unique condition of the "locked-in syndrome," the mind stays alive but cannot communicate. However, the electrical patterns, cerebral blood flow, oxygen usage of that brain can be determined. When coupled with eyelid movement, these signs prove that the person is still there.

[2] The brain died within minutes of the cessation of other vital organs, or, if the brain died first, the rest of the body soon followed.

[3] Of course, consciousness is not necessarily an on/off switch. Sometimes there are low levels of brain activity within the common situation known as a coma. And among the profoundly retarded, one can find those who lack the familiar expressions of the human personality or soul. They may be only marginally self-conscious, unable to communicate, and fairly unresponsive. So have we started down a slippery slope that will one day exclude all these people? I do not think so. Retarded and demented persons *are* conscious, as well as those in a reversible coma, which can now be determined with considerable reliability.

[4] Robert J. Lifton, *The Nazi Doctors* (New York: Basic Books, Inc., 1986), p. 63.

[5] Dave and Neta Jackson, *Glimpses of Glory* (Elgin, Illinois: Brethren Press, 1987), p. 266.

[6] D. Elton Trueblood, *General Philosophy* (New York: Harper and Row, Publishers, 1963), p. 278.

[7] Ibid., pp. 278–279.

[8] Ibid., pp. 279–280.

CHAPTER SEVEN

What I'd Want For Myself

C ompare theory and reality in your own life. Ever notice a difference? I find the same in my own life! So it's quite natural for people to wonder what I'd *really* want for myself when I go through the dying process. We all think that if a doctor could choose how to die, he or she would chose the most peaceful and painless way. Well, I cannot promise you the last word on the dying process. Besides, I couldn't guarantee an ideal death anyhow, even for myself. But if I've been observant during my 25 years as a physician, then my wishes should be informed by at least the compassion of self-interest—and hopefully much more.

To share my own wishes, first I would like to tell you what have been the most helpful concepts I have learned as I have taken care of many dying patients. Then I'll outline several different physical scenarios of how I might die and what I'd like under those circumstances and why. In this way you too can walk in my shoes and thereby better tackle this difficult subject for yourself.

Finally, we will look at the idea of "living wills," those legal documents prepared before a life-threatening crisis to communicate a person's wishes should life-support decisions arise.

The Art of Dying

1. Preparation for death. Shortly after receiving my M.D. degree and while still an intern at the university hospital, I helped care for several seriously ill patients whose deaths their families had not expected. When the patient died, I followed what I had learned in training and began telling the family by pronouncing the death first. But from the moment that I said that their loved one had died, they stopped hearing anything else that I said. So I couldn't console them. I wondered how I would react to the news if one of my close friends or family members died. This taught me to prepare people before I said, "He's dead." And guess what? Preparation prevented the excessively overwhelming reaction that had paralyzed the previously unprepared survivors.

2. People aren't possessions. As a result of those early experiences with death, I decided that I needed to keep in mind the fact that everyone has to die and, therefore, no family member or friend is mine to keep but only to care for and enjoy for a season. This truth will help me let them go when the time comes. This doesn't mean that I cannot love them deeply. Rather, I now have learned how to hold them even closer than before, and not take them for granted.

3. The school of life. In this same way, I learned the great value that life has, not only for today but as training for tomorrow. Life must have been designed to change and mature me. If this were not so, then the circumstances of life that buffet, shove, and squeeze me would be cruel manipulations with no redeeming value. The problems of life would all be outside me, a picture from which I am detached. Instead, I believe life is a drama in which I am a participant, involved and affected by the drama itself. For this reason I consider the purpose of life itself to provide all the learning opportunities that I need for me to become a mature human being.

The benefit of life's experiences occurs for me to learn how to live life better and become a better person. They help me to personally grow beyond what I could accomplish with human help. Yet on a higher plane life's experiences lead me into encounters with my Maker where I can experience God's faithfulness and love for me. The profit I gain from life's experiences includes learning to see life from God's perspective, a point from which I can now serve humankind to the glory of God.

4. The need for companions. If I am so fortunate as to remain alert so that I can spend meaningful time with other people, I would like to have some people go through my dying experience with me. I could benefit from people who would be faithful and trustworthy, who would continue visiting until I die. I am well aware that it will be difficult for those people, but I also believe that it will be profitable for them. After all, the essence of life is found in relationships.

5. Putting my life into perspective. In addition to companionship, there is great benefit in honest dialogue that helps the dying person put life into perspective. This must involve someone who is willing to talk about more than the weather, current events, or their own problems. The person doesn't have to have any answers. Perhaps we could discover many of the answers together. But since I will be weak and tired, I'll need the person to spend a little of his or her strength in discussing the issues. Here are some of the questions I would like help facing:

- Do I have to die now? (This should be a sober review of my condition and what my options are.)
- Am I facing my condition and the finality of death or am I denying it, living in the fantasy that this isn't really happening to me? (Facing the reality of death does not mean the same as passively giving up. There's much to fight for in seeking the courage to be able to exalt Christ through the process.)
- What has been the meaning of my life? What has it counted for? What has been the central theme of my life? What other threads have I woven through my life? On the basis of how I've lived, who has been my Lord? (Pat answers are

useless here.)

- What has the process of my disease or condition meant to me and my family? Have there been emotional and spiritual changes for better or worse?
- Is my dying consistent with the life that I have lived? That is, can I respect myself as much in my dying as in my living?
- How am I treating those around me while I'm dying?
- Are there guilts or resentments that need to be settled? Are there relationships that need to be mended?

6. Stories of those who have gone before. A great deal of encouragement and peace can be communicated through reviewing how others have faced death and suffering. This might include stories of Christian martyrs as reported in *Fox's Book of Martyrs* or *Martyrs Mirror* and a variety of contemporary stories, including Christians who have died from more natural causes.

7. Providing distractions. Though I must face my condition, don't let me become obsessed with it and its pain. Point out the joy of the other things in the world, particularly those that affect my family and friends. Bring me enthusiasm for life each day you visit. And always bring me a smile and laughter. Share a few jokes with me. Listen to my jokes and let's laugh together.

8. Reading Scripture. If I am unable to read, or if it tires me too much, you could do me a great service by reading Scripture. Even if I can read easily, your sharing it with me would be especially valuable. Not only will I experience peace as I put my affairs in this life in order and into perspective, but I will gain eagerness for the life to come as I meditate on the Lord. Many of the biblical passages we read will remind us of experiences that we've had in life. Then we can share with each other how God worked in us and for us. Finally, we can each contribute what God did through us. This will make my dying a time of rejoicing and celebration.

How we encounter life-threatening conditions varies greatly

from a physical perspective. Many times the question of using a life-support system doesn't arise. But here are a variety of possible scenarios where it might and my preferences for each.

Terminal But Alert

If I am in a terminal condition but mentally alert, I want to be part of the decision-making process concerning my treatment and care. Why do I insist on this? Because I am responsible for my life, and the choices I make are part of what makes me human. Even in the dying process, I am accountable for the person that I am, and I want to make the best choices and use of my time.

If a particular treatment will *likely* extend my life significantly, I would probably like to have it. If its value is questionable, I'd rather be made as comfortable as possible. I'd rather use my body's resources and energies to live out my remaining days in relationship with others rather than in a struggle for more time on earth.

Remember that I have dedicated my life to God. He provides my strength and extends to me an inner comfort and peace that passes all understanding. This peace with God comes from having been justified by faith through our Lord Jesus Christ. His peace has been so deep and pure that it has abided in me through every situation of my life, even after my five-hour operation which produced the worst pain that I've ever experienced. Therefore, I want to spend my remaining days communing with Him instead of striving for an extension of time on this earth. Let me be as alert to Him as possible. Then I want time to be with people, particularly my loved ones, as we work through my dying every inch of the way.

Heart Attack or Stroke

If I have a heart attack or a stroke and someone can give me CPR, please do so. Take me to the hospital and try to resuscitate me. If I survive, great. If, however, I fail to regain consciousness, follow the guidelines described later in this list for determining and responding to a permanent loss of consciousness. When my brain dies, my mind and soul depart, so release my body too.

Conscious But on Life Support

If I am resuscitated but require life-support systems, continue using them until I have recovered enough to live without them. In that case, life support will have prolonged my life, and I will have more time to serve God and my fellow humans. I will be grateful.

On the other hand, if my condition deteriorates and the prognosis means that I will never recover enough to live without life supports, continue using them as necessary, but don't add any new ones. If I am alert and can communicate with you, I'll tell you when I've had enough. If I am incompetent, don't add anything to my treatment that would prolong my dying—no operations, no antibiotics, no CPR! Let that second intruder bring my death.

No matter what care you give me or don't give me, please do not abandon me. Your human contact has more worth than anything else you can give me. And your presence, even if you don't know what to say, will help me bear my burden.

Unconsciousness after Anesthesia

If I have an operation and do not regain consciousness but develop a permanent loss of consciousness, follow the procedures outlined below (see "Permanent Loss of Consciousness"). However, if I have sufficient retention of consciousness to be aware of myself and others, then provide the appropriate level of care for my condition for the rest of my life.

If I'm not alert enough to communicate adequately with my family and friends and am in a terminal state, then do not resuscitate me again if I have a cardiac arrest. If I have a major infection or other life-threatening condition, do not treat it.

Let me die a natural death. If I am not conscious enough to tell you to treat the condition that will bring about my death sooner than the original terminal condition, don't treat it.

I am ready to die. I have worked through my own death as well as I can without actually and imminently facing it. I have been saved by faith in Christ Jesus. Therefore, I have died to sin, the wages of which is death, and am alive in Christ and will be resurrected by Him who raised Jesus Christ from the dead. So I am looking forward to my new life in God's presence: this is my hope. After all, I've lived in that new life for many years already, so I know it's real.

Permanent Loss of Consciousness

If I have an ailment or injury that leaves me permanently comatose, and that diagnosis has been established accurately on clinical grounds and by pulsed Doppler ultrasound (PDU) measurements and/or positron emission tomographic (PET) scans of regional cerebral blood flow and glucose metabolism (as discussed in Chapter 3), pull the plug! If my brain stem still functions and my body continues to breathe on its own, remove the IV fluids and feeding tube as well. Do this even if some residual cortical electrical activity registers on the EEG that causes the body to make inappropriate and meaningless movements. If I have permanently lost consciousness, I have already died, so let my body quit too.

If there are any healthy organs in my body that could prolong *life* for another person, I'd be happy to donate them. Instead of pulling the plug as soon as my diagnosis has been firmly established, proceed with the transplantation—however long that may take—then pull the plug. Don't wait until my organs die and become useless.

Dementia

If I develop dementia but am self-conscious, I would like the basic goal of my treatment to be aimed at improving my quality of life. Don't just decide that people in my state need this or that but consider who I am, who I have been, and what I might think is helpful to me.

My family will know enough about me that their guidance may be trusted in this regard. Choose treatments, activities, foods, and medications on the basis of what might lower my level of distress and what would allow me to be more of the person I used to be.

Give me a thorough workup and treat those things that might decrease my dementia. Reassess my condition frequently enough to evaluate the effectiveness of various treatments. If a treatment becomes no longer effective, stop using it. Try something else that would be more appropriate. When I am dying, keep me comfortable, but don't spend time trying to prolong my dying. Instead, give me tender, loving care rather than a mechanical existence.

Excruciating Pain

The dying process might be quite painful and agonizing; I might even talk about death—of dying sooner than my disease would kill me—but I do not mean that I want to commit suicide or that anyone else should kill me even if that may seem to be merciful.

I know what terrible, agonizing pain is. I have stood at the bedside of a number of people who have suffered from excruciating, tormenting pain and watched them twist and groan to find a position that might ease the pain for a few moments. Some required intravenous morphine in high doses every hour or two around the clock and still did not find adequate control of their pain. Others were unable to lie down to sleep, walk, or move because of the excessive pain it caused.

I remember what horrible pain I had after the five-hour operation I endured to remove my gallbladder. I felt like a Mack truck had hit me. I couldn't believe anything could hurt so much. Yet the pain forms only one side of the reality. The other side contains life's meaning and value that pain cannot destroy. As Gordon W. Allport, a professor of psychology at Harvard University, has said, "Life becomes intolerable only to those who feel that there is nothing more for which they can live and to which they can aspire."

As a physician, I am sure that there is much in life that can reduce unbearable pain. And as a Christian I remain convinced, like the Apostle Paul, that God is the God of compassion and all comfort. He can and will provide whatever I need not only to cope with but to transcend my agony. And that actual dependency on Him assures me that I should not trust in myself or other humans but in God, who raised Jesus Christ from the dead, in whom I've set my hope, and who will deliver me through resurrection to eternal life.

Living through my dying process and working through its pain will be my final act of trust in God. I have been practicing that trust throughout life, and I want my dying to express my greatest trust in Him. He has saved me from my sin and over the years I have encountered His Spirit working through me and through others. In responding to Him, I have gained a joy and peace that provides a dignity far more validating than any pain I have experienced can nullify. He has been so faithful that I believe I can entrust my dying to Him also. Furthermore, I have seen His faithfulness in a number of dying people who have testified to His unwavering trustworthiness in sustaining their dignity.

What About Living Wills?

In recent years the specter of being connected to some machine that prolongs the dying process has given rise to the idea of "living wills" which declare in advance a patient's desire to not have the dying process artificially prolonged. These have been created in an effort to avoid prolonged and expensive court battles over the question of what should be done with an incompetent patient.

The Society for the Right to Die has offered the model on page 113.

LIVING WILL DECLARATION

To My Family, Doctors, and All Those Concerned with My Care,

I, _____ , being of sound mind, make this statement as a directive to be followed if I become unable to participate in decisions regarding my medical care.

If I should be in an incurable or irreversible mental or physical condition with no reasonable expectation of recovery, I direct my attending physician to withhold or withdraw treatment that merely prolongs my dying. I further direct that treatment be limited to measures to keep me comfortable and to relieve pain.

These directions express my legal right to refuse treatment. Therefore, I expect my family, doctors, and everyone concerned with my care to regard themselves as legally and morally bound to act in accord with my wishes, and in so doing to be free from any legal liability for having followed my directions.

I especially do not want:_____

Other instructions/comments:_____

By means of instructions at the side of the form, it is recommended that undesired treatment such as "cardiac resuscitation, mechanical respiration, artificial feeding/ fluids by tubes" be identified after: "I especially do not want." "Other instructions" might include requests for things the person *does* want, such as dying at home.

The form then concludes with a place for a "Proxy Designation Clause" (sometimes known as a "durable power of attorney") and signatures of the person and two witnesses.

Also, the Society provides other forms that use the actual wording of the various statutes in the 38 states (plus the District of Columbia) that have passed what is popularly known as right-to-die or living-will legislation.[1] The wording varies slightly from state to state primarily in terms of the witness requirements, though the laws in some states, such as Oklahoma, do not include a provision for withdrawing medication and sustenance for incompetent patients.

According to their stated goal, "The Society works for the right to die with dignity. It seeks to protect the individual's right to control treatment decisions at the end of life, including the right to refuse unwanted medical procedures, that can only prolong the dying process. It pursues this objective through activities in three general areas: educational, legislative, and judicial." When questioned, Shirley Neitlich, the Society's public information representative said, "We favor allowing people to die, not causing them to die. We have no official position on active euthanasia."

Concerns About Living Wills

I have three concerns relative to living wills.

First, I believe that extreme care must be taken to limit the withholding or withdrawal of life-sustaining measures to only those patients with neocortical *death* or in the *actual process of dying*. The form supplied by the Society for the Right to Die seems far too broad in stipulating "an incurable or irreversible mental or physical condition with no reasonable expectation of recovery." That does not seem to require the condition to be even terminal.

Second, care should also be taken so that senility, dementia (which are often "irreversible mental conditions"), or other quality-of-life questions cannot in any way be construed as a cause for withdrawing care. Some of these conditions are not fatal in themselves. Only when a patient enters into the actual process of dying should that process not be prolonged.

Third, some advocates of living wills may not have taken an

official position favoring euthanasia, but they do constitute a powerful lobbying and educational movement that ultimately may pave the road for the approval of euthanasia. I would feel much more comfortable if the Society for the Right to Die and other such groups became vigorously *opposed* to euthanasia and took pains to define *death* in contrast to the *quality of life*.

But that gets into the subject of the next chapter: Is there a slippery slope, and what are the dangers of sliding down it?

Notes

[1] Case law prevails in the 12 states without specific legislation. The case law in New Jersey, for instance, is more liberal than the statutes passed in most states that have dealt with the subject through legislation.

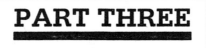

PART THREE

The
Forces for
Death

CHAPTER EIGHT

The Slippery Slope to Euthanasia

If we lower our ethic from "do everything possible to sustain life as long as possible," aren't we opening a Pandora's box of conditional decision-making that will ultimately lead to euthanasia, possibly even mandatory euthanasia?

Some concerned people fear exactly that. And there is cause for such concern. Except when the Holy Spirit has invaded history to convict of sin and stir revival, moral decay seems to be the most common course of society. Even the advancements in civilization are often either the product of spiritual revival or just a reorganization of power that seems to correct some evils but often at the expense of encouraging others.

The Slippery Slope Theory

Our moral decay has taken giant steps in the recent past. Most people shiver when they look at the consequences, and yet this same decay ironically results from our compulsion to turn to technology to solve our moral problems rather than turning to God. But the more we rely on technology to solve our moral problems—of which life support represents but one—the more we become morally paralyzed. Why? Because technology is morally neutral; it does not care whether we use it to destroy all the life on our planet or grow food for hungry people. It cannot advise us.

And yet because technology can sometimes be used to solve problems, it entices us to rely on it unquestioningly, even though it produces an equal number of problems. We think a technological problem must have a technological solution. The result has been called the slippery slope phenomenon. Its progress might be diagramed as follows:

Into relative moral equilibrium
technology introduces a *dilemma:*

If we *can* do this,
then why not do that?
If that is *OK,*
why not this other?

If an outside reference point
is not consulted, the conclusion can be *immorality.*

The slippery slope affects us in subtle increments which in themselves seem not only harmless but often as helpful individual steps. Yet once we take the first step, we may be halfway down the slope to the next step. By measuring each succeeding step only against the previous one—instead of the original ground—we can end up at the bottom in a morass of tragic immorality without even realizing how we got to a place that would have shocked us at first.

Abortion, a Contemporary Example

Those concerned about the slippery slope in the arena of medical ethics have only to point to the recent history of abortion to find a dramatic example. Here acquiescing at one level led with surprising quickness to something far worse than anyone ever envisioned at the outset. Technology introduced the dilemma: "*If we can* actually abort a fetus easily and safely, *then why not* do it for women facing a life-threatening pregnancy?" Next the victims of rape and incest were included in technology's answer to a tragic pregancy: Why should these victims have to endure the trauma of bearing an unwanted child? The supporting arguments soon focused on the problem of other "unwanted pregancies": Why should a pregnant teenager be forced to disrupt her whole life by carrying to term the product of one brief mistake? If the rich can get abortions out of state or out of the country, why should we discriminate against the poor, forcing them to use dangerous back-alley services? Why should women have to bear the consequences for sexual encounters? And finally, why shouldn't women have as much control over their own bodies as men do?

By the time abortion on demand was secured for the first trimester, technology had made it relatively safe for the mother at later stages: "*If it's okay* to do early abortions, *then why not* later ones now that they are safe?"

Soon abortions became common during the second and even third trimester—well past the time when some premature babies could survive. Now, with abortion considered a universal right by many, it has become a common means of birth control for some.

The slippery slope has already created some disasters in logical thinking. A high school girl, for instance, cannot be given any medical treatment—even an aspirin by the school nurse—without her parents' permission. But most states do not require parental consent or even knowledge if their daughter requests an abortion. And although women can have their unborn infants aborted at will, drunken drivers who have caused unborn infants to die in the womb have been charged with murder.

In 1980, California became the first state to uphold a malpractice suit for "wrongful life" when Philis and Hyam Curlender charged that Bio-Science Laboratories falsely assured them that neither of them carried the gene of Tay-Sachs disease, a fatal neurological disorder peculiar to Eastern European Jews. Their daughter, Shauna, was born with the disease. Since then more than 150 wrongful-life suits and a equal number of wrongful-birth suits have been decided in 21 states.[1] Many of these suits are based on the notion that the parents could have aborted their handicapped child if they had been adequately advised.

Clark Forsythe, staff counsel for Americans United for Life, says, "The implication is that ... *any* handicapped life is wrongful. . . . These suits foster the most blatant form of discrimination against the handicapped imaginable. . . . This is compassion as contempt."[2] (Fortunately, six states have passed legislation prohibiting suits like this.)

We are still sliding down the slippery slope. Sharon Sheppard, writing in *Family Life Today* magazine, says that Surgeon General Koop has identified a shocking rise in the incidents of infanticide in this country. He found a number of people choosing not to treat severely handicapped newborns. For instance, some let infants with Down's syndrome simply starve to death.[3]

And where will it end? Sheppard thinks an early prediction may soon come to pass:

In May 1973, just four months after the Supreme Court's decision to legalize abortion on demand, *Time* magazine quoted scientist and Nobel Prize winner James D. Watson's suggestion that perhaps parents as a routine matter ought to have a few days to decide whether they want to keep their child. Watson said, "If a child were not declared alive until three days after birth, then parents could be allowed the choice only a few are given under the present system. The doctor could allow the child to die if the parents so chose and save a lot of misery and suffering."[4]

The Slippery Slope and the Life-Support Dilemma

Is there a cause to fear that the life-support dilemma is perched on this kind of a slippery slope? Could it happen here also? Well, already our modern technological care of patients has too often been at the expense of human compassion and comfort. That has also resulted in a *new* prospect for us all: the possibility of being forced to endure an unnatural, lingering dying process and/or have our bodies kept functioning long after we die. The accompanying sense of helplessness and loss of meaning has caused people to demand their right to privacy. They want protection from such measures and the opportunity to exercise their self-determination.

These are legitimate concerns.

But the Hemlock Society and other groups dedicated to euthanasia are exploiting this dilemma as the perfect time to gain public acceptance of their objectives. And those objectives are at the bottom of a very ugly slope. The proposal for the Humane and Dignified Death Act already includes provisions forbidding family members from being able to stop a killing, insuring that the executioners would be free from prosecution, and a declared search for a way to bring euthanasia to the mentally incompetent (who by definition can have no active choice in the matter).

In her article "Deadly Mercy," Melinda Delahoyde suggests that the tactics of the Hemlock Society are as follows:

> [At this time] very few people believe that someone who is not dying should be starved to death or helped to commit suicide because they no longer have a "meaningful life." [Yet] these are the real goals of the euthanasia forces. But knowing that the American public will not accept this kind of forced killing, they hide their true goals behind cases where someone who is already dying simply wants to be left alone.[5]

"Freedom of choice" is a key theme in the euthanasia movement, but Surgeon General Koop warns: "What is voluntary euthanasia now, you can bet your bottom dollar will be mandatory euthanasia in days ahead."[6]

Why is this the likely conclusion of slipping to the bottom of this slope? Because if the decision between life and death remains based upon quality-of-life questions, then when those qualities cease, the person is really "better off dead," *whether they admit it or not*. When someone is considered useless to themselves and a burden to society, the "right to die" will become the "duty to die." What justification would they have for continuing to consume resources that others might use better?

So, what are the options?

The Option to Acquiesce

Those who are overwhelmed by the dilemma will accept the inevitability of the steps down the slope.

The first step is evaluating the worth of life according to the quality of life.

The second step accepts the notion that there is no difference between the right to reject life-sustaining treatment and active euthanasia. (Therefore, why not allow the latter?)

The third step claims that if competent people have the right to die (through active euthanasia), the incompetent deserve the same.

That process brings one to the bottom of the slope where we would be killing the "useless" and unwanted, even against their will. But even more terrifying is this: those who have the power—and in any society the power is invested in someone—decide who are the useless and unwanted.

The Option to Retreat

Convinced that if they yield to making any decisions about life and death, society will inevitably slip to the bottom of the slope, some people propose withdrawing from the dilemma by making every effort technically possible to preserve life, by insisting on never withdrawing life support, and by rejecting any form of a living will or durable power of attorney.

But the ground to which they retreat is indefensible. This

dilemma will not go away. The flood of new technology will rise to erode any temporary refuge they may reach. Today's life-support machines will soon seem as primitive as a wooden plow, and bodies or partial bodies or synthetically grown parts will become sustainable for years. Elderly people will be suspended—possibly in pain—indefinitely.

Certainly in every case we have the risk of an error. Wisdom calls us to err on the side of keeping someone alive longer than necessary rather than risk killing them prematurely. Consider the magnitude of this problem. As previously noted, the American Medical Association estimates that medical institutions artificially sustain approximately 10,000 permanently unconscious individuals. Indeed, even today, every elderly person who does not succumb to a quick death (which cannot be medically intervened) faces the potential of having his or her life artificially prolonged. The potential of our technological nightmare has got to end somewhere, and the only way to end it lies in courageously making some decisions concerning it.

Life-Respecting Assertions

A better option than either acquiescing or retreating is to make life-respecting assertions consistent with God's Word. Such a solid foundation is not in danger of slipping or being eroded.

1. All human life must be defended. Regardless of the quality of one's life, each person became a "living soul" as the result of a gift from God. No one has the right to take that gift from another or discard his or her own gift of life.

2. Not all "life" is human life. Bodies from which the human spirit has departed do not constitute human life and do not have to be protected as human life. To the degree that we can determine with certainty when a permanent loss of consciousness has taken place (the death of the neocortex), we may regard the remaining body as not constituting human life.

Some may wonder whether defining death is, in itself, a compromising first step down the slippery slope. Yes, that will continue as a problem that we must guard against. Therefore, I'd like to spend a little time on it.

Perhaps the best approach would be to take another look at abortion.

For centuries Western civilization accepted the understanding that taking the life of the unborn was to kill a human being. But when modern technology made it safe and simple to perform abortions, there developed a pressure to use that technology—first of all to provide an alternative to back-alley abortionists. Our technological advances had been so striking and helpful in many areas of life that people began to look at technology as a part of the natural order of life. "If we can do it, it can't be wrong. Besides, look how easily we can solve those previously impossible problems."

Suddenly the fetus became the problem. And since technology could quickly remove the problem, why not use it and end the "problem" for many women. In order to justify such an action, society has to focus on the fetus as the problem, the impurity to be removed. Since technology is amoral (neither moral or immoral) no one, it was thought, would suffer psychologically, ethically, or spiritually.

In addition to this, the proabortion forces set out to dispute the *humanness* of the fetus. Since no one could prove technologically when a fetus became an actual living human being, the fetus was declared not to be a human being yet. And if the fetus was not a human being, then it was not immoral to destroy it, so the reasoning went.

Now back to the problem of the definition of death. We are not suggesting that what has always been considered human should now be called nonhuman. What we are saying is that the technology of life-support systems has shown us beyond the shadow of a doubt that a person whose cerebral cortex is dead is no longer a human being, even if a machine keeps the rest of his body alive for weeks or months or even years.

A body which contains a dead cortex has no potential, *ever,* of becoming a human being again in any sense of the word. The mind and soul, those essential elements of being human, are gone forever. But in the case of the fetus or even the embryo, there was nothing until conception but two individual cells with no inherent potential of being human as long as they remained apart.

But when the sperm fertilized the egg, a complete human being was started. From that time on, nothing is added to that growing human but food, oxygen, removal of waste, and time. Just think, the full potential of an adult human being—an Einstein, a Ruth, a Mozart, another Apostle Paul, or the mother of a great family. The body with a dead cortex has no potential for being human.

Therefore, I do not believe we are on the slippery slope. We are not *redefining* death. The point here is that in the process of dying, the cerebral cortex dies when the human being dies and vice versa, not when all the rest of his body dies. Only machines have significantly separated the death of the cerebral cortex from that of the rest of the body. I'm suggesting that we return to that general perspective as our baseline. Then, we may ask whether there is a hopeful reason to hook up the machines in an effort to prolong life. For many there will be such a reason, but not for all.

3. People are free to meet their natural dates with death. Refusing life-sustaining treatment *is* distinct from active euthanasia precisely because the first accepts a date with death that God allows, while the second creates an artificial date, taking life and death into one's own hands. This distinction frees us not to *have* to do everything possible to cling to life for a few more days, weeks, or months. When the Lord opens the door, we may walk through to be with Him.

4. True "death with dignity" requires courage. "No pain, no gain," says the athlete, and most of us know we're better off going to the dentist than not. No one welcomes or invites pain and suffering, but there are some things more important than avoiding it. One of the characteristics of human maturity lies in the ability to delay gratification and rise above the Pavlovian reaction of an animal. In the context of the life-support dilemma, behaving in a morally responsible manner—even if it hurts—requires one of those mature choices. If making morally responsible choices means we must accept pain in this life, the great reward we anticipate in the next life will be Christ's commendation: "Well done, thou good and faithful servant."

Nonetheless facing that pain often requires more courage than we think we can muster. But God has never promised to stockpile our courage in advance. Instead, in the very moment of the trial God's provision becomes sufficient. First Corinthians 10:13 promises: "No temptation has seized you except what is common to man. And God is faithful; He will not let you be tempted beyond what you can bear. But when you are tempted, He will also provide a way out so that you can stand up under it."

(Lest anyone misunderstand the "way out" as condoning euthanasia, the context of 1 Corinthians 9 and 10 emphasizes faithfulness in adversity in contrast to weak self-indulgence. The next verses, 14-17, explicitly challenge us to embrace the cup of Christ's suffering in the context of the bread of His body—possibly a suggestion that strength and relief will most often come through relationships.)

Dying with this confidence—to glorify God in the face of our enemy, death—is true "death with dignity" that can never be achieved through a bottle of pills and the desertion of our post.

Suicide is wrong not just because God is supposed to decide when death is to come to anyone but because it is an outright statement that God is not sufficient for the problems of life. In other words, it declares that God made a mistake in designing the world, or that He is not sovereign or master of it all. It is putting the creature before the Creator, which is the basis of the sin.

5. *Self-determination and relationships compose the most life-respecting supports.* When someone faces death, we need to affirm his right of self-determination within the bounds of morality, and we need to maintain a relationship with him as

he goes through his valley. In some cases a relationship may be secure enough to entrust it with the authority to carry out another's will even when that person cannot express it for himself or herself.

Some people speak of such a "durable power of attorney" in alarmist terms: "This gives someone else sweeping power to make health care decisions for you if you become incompetent. In the event you are ill this person would have the power to decide if you live or die"[7]—as though anyone would give that authority to some hostile stranger.

But if you do become incompetent, then by definition someone else *will* be making those decisions for you. This forces the question, "Who?" The real strangers in such an instance would be the courts and hospital bureaucracies applying impersonal rules in a what is hoped would be an impartial way. I would certainly prefer to trust my spouse, a loving son or daughter, pastor, or Christian friend who knows me well; they would have a much greater chance of choosing exactly what I would want. Of course, one must be concerned about who receives this power over our care, but it is far more Christian to cultivate such trustworthy relationships between people than to fall back on the protection of the state.

I believe the above five assertions will not slide down the euthanasist's slippery slope but will provide a solid ethical foundation to meet the technology of today and face the developments to come in the foreseeable future.

Notes

[1] Gregg Levoy, "Body," Omni, October 1987, p. 30.
[2] David Neff, "Compassion as Contempt," *Christianity Today,* October 16, 1987, p. 15.
[3] Sharon Sheppard, "The Surgeon General Speaks Out On the Right to Live, the Right to Die," *Family Life Today,* May/June 1985, p. 35.
[4] Ibid., p. 36.
[5] Melinda Delahoyde, "Deadly Mercy," in *Pastoral Renewal,* Vol. 10, No. 7, February 1986, p. 112.
[6] Sheppard, ·p. 36.
[7] Delahoyde, p. 112.

CHAPTER NINE

The Physician as Healer/Killer

istorical records indicate that for nearly 4,000 years physicians have taken oaths to practice medicine for the benefit of their patients' lives. Some of these recorded oaths include the *Code of Hammurabi* of the Babylonians, the *Oath of Hippocrates* in the Greek culture, and the *Code of Medical Ethics* of Dr. Thomas Percival at the beginning of the 1800s.[1] Over those four millennia the cumulative ethic for all physicians was: "I will use treatment to help the sick according to my ability and judgment, but never with a view to injury and wrongdoing. Neither will I administer a poison to anyone when asked to do so, nor will I suggest such a course."

And yet, still ringing in my ears are the words of the Hemlock Society: "The Hemlock Society announces the publication of the Humane and Dignified Death Act which will permit a physician to end the life of a dying patient upon the competent request of the patient."

Dr. Robert Jay Lifton, who has studied the subject of death and dying from Japan to Germany, says in his book *The Nazi Doctors:*

Psychologically speaking, nothing is darker or more menacing, or harder to accept, than the participation of physicians in mass murder. However technicized or commercial the modern physician may have become, he or she is still supposed to be a healer—and one responsible to a tradition of healing, which all cultures revere and depend upon. Knowledge that the doctor has joined the killers adds a grotesque dimension to the perception that "this world is not this world."[2]

Why Doctor-assisted Suicide?

As a physician and a healer, I can attest to the schizophrenia of being asked to also become one who kills. So why are doctors being enlisted in the grim task of helping people die? The Hemlock Society claims that there are too many "botched" attempts when a person or friend or relative tries to do it themselves, and, therefore, someone who is knowledgeable must help them.

In some circumstances incapacitated people literally do not have the means or the ability to kill themselves. But there are other inhibitors. Each year in this country thousands of physically healthy people attempt suicide and fortunately fail. In many cases, there is reason to believe that their *will to live* actually won out over their despair and subconsciously guided them to an ineffective suicide attempt. Yes, they reached a point of such mental agony that they took a bottle of pills, slashed their wrists, or jumped from a window, but out of some hidden ambivalence they called for help at the last moment or chose an action that was not reasonably certain to fulfill their objective.

What if we offered all those people a surefire way to succeed? I know many people who have recovered from their psychological problems who would be dead today if someone would have helped them when they said they wanted to kill themselves.

Of course, euthanasists are currently focusing only on individuals who are suffering at the end stage of life. But I think the principle has not changed. God has placed within us a very strong will to live, and though we may despair of life, that will to live inhibits us from ending it all before God's time.

Even relatives and friends hesitate to do the deed for a suffering loved one. If they were so certain that it was the loving thing to do, why would they require a third party—a physician—to put their loved one out of his or her misery? They have the desire to help, the request, the privacy, and the available materials; and it would serve the patient's desire for self-determination, all seemingly in the patient's best interest. Could it be the moral repulsiveness of the act of killing someone?

Might the love relationship itself make it so difficult for a relative to help? Then maybe that same love relationship means more than death itself. Maybe the dying person needs love in greater measure rather than a premature death.

How could it be any easier for a physician to commit murder than a lay person or other professional? Because of our training, the oaths we take, and our deep commitment to the preservation of life, committing murder would be extremely hard for most physicians. For instance, Dr. Lester Martin taught me the surgical care of children at the Cincinnati Children's Hospital as a part of my surgical training at the University of Cincinnati. And now sixteen years later, I still remember how Dr. Martin taught us to stay at the bedside of very sick children without taking a break, except to go to the bathroom, until the threat of death passed and the child began to recover.

But given this great antagonism between healing and killing, is it possible for healers to become killers? Unfortunately, yes. The reasons come as no great mystery. First, doctors are human and have within them the seeds to kill or commit any other sin. Second, sooner or later the collective requirements of society become the ethics of its physicians.

I want to look more closely at each of these dynamics as we consider what it might mean to ask our doctors to become killers.

Doctors Are Only Human

Do you remember the case of Wyman Garrett that I mentioned in Chapter 1? He was the New Jersey doctor who pleaded no contest to charges of gross malpractice and other improprieties involving 40 patients. His attorney offered as a defense for his behavior the fact that he had been unable to discern between good and evil after performing 2,700 late-stage abortions; as a result he had suffered intense emotional "burnout."

Was Garrett unique? Or was he an example of the loss of perspective that can happen to any physician who compromises his role as healer by also working as a killer?

No One Can Serve Two Masters

Jesus said, "No one can serve two masters. Either he will hate the one and love the other, or he will be devoted to the one and despise the other. You cannot serve both God and Money" (Matt. 6:24). The same applies for any other opposing forces that compete for our allegiance. Physicians must devote their full thinking and commitment to honoring life and the health of their patients. If they think, plan, and execute actions designed for terminating life, they lose something of their keen sense of promoting life, their judgment in using their skills toward that end, and their moral strength.

When a physician practices active euthanasia, the very moral ground that constitutes his excellence as a physician is blunted and slowly but surely lost. At some point that physician turns away from a basic stance of healing to one in which killing—more efficiently, less traumatically—becomes paramount.

Not only do the finest points of the physician's judgment decline as he or she indulges in active killing (for whatever reason), but various psychological changes also occur. As this change happens it's sometimes hard to tell whether it happened before the killings and set the stage allowing the doctor to practice euthanasia, or after he started killings and occurred as a reaction to them.

How does that change occur? Once one starts thinking in terms of killing, one begins seeing patients with the same thought in mind. It becomes an option that subtly injects itself into every situation. For example, the insidious way death as an option takes over one's thinking can be seen in the comments of Dr. Howard Caplan, who practices geriatrics at 30 nursing homes. In his article "It's Time We Helped Patients Die," he shares the following anecdotal perspectives, seemingly oblivious of how he's become preoccupied with seeing his patients through the eyes of the grim reaper:

> "Well, I wonder if Mrs. M. would be better off dead."
>
> "Wow, Mr. J. has little left of his personality. I wonder if he could talk clearly and coherently, would he want euthanasia. I think so."
>
> "And oh yes, Mrs. A. over there has to have help often to do the basic activities of her life. She's sure getting older and seems to be failing more as of late. If I were to ask her if she would like to die now instead of dying slowly and be so embarrassed about it, she'd probably tell me: 'I'm ready to go. My bags are packed. Help me.'"
>
> "And if I thought a particular patient was a candidate and her son who only keeps contact by telephone with the nursing home said, 'Well, I can't really get away, Doctor, but I violently disagree,' my answer would be, 'Well, not violently enough. Everyone here can see what shape your mother's in. We're quite sure what she'd want if she could tell us, and we're going to help her.'"[3]

The Danger of Abuse

As the idea of killing develops, the request arises for more authority for physicians so that they can make decisions as they see fit on behalf of their patients. But doctors are just as susceptible to abusing their authority as anyone else. And the danger grows by using a "successful" treatment indiscriminately or for personal gain.

In medical circles we call the indiscriminate use of drugs the "shotgun" approach. When a new, very powerful drug becomes available, some doctors use it to treat not only the disease it's specifically designed for, but every disease to which it might be applied.

For example, Chloromycetin, a very powerful but extremely effective antibiotic, was used for every illness possible, especially minor sore throats, etc. The rationale focused on its safety and effectiveness. So why not use it to nip all infections in the bud? Suddenly, a few years later we found that Chloromycetin caused a deadly side effect: it destroyed the bone marrow of a small number of patients. Now we can't use it without fear of a lawsuit.

The Hemlock Society's proposal has very few safeguards against abuse. The request of the patient and the concurrence of two doctors make up all that would be required. The family could not interfere.

Unfortunately, there are occasionally unscrupulous physicians who—for reasons too diverse to list—might secure someone's permission ("request") for euthanasia in pressurized ways. Some anti-euthanasists place their strongest emphasis on this aspect of possible abuse. They conjure up horror stories of greedy heirs bribing a doctor to give a struggling old woman a lethal injection so that they can divide the inheritance.

Crimes can occur under any circumstances. We shouldn't make them more convenient, so this potential for criminal abuse should not be overlooked. But greater concern to me lies in the tendency for people in all the caring professions to play God—to think, as did Dr. Howard Caplan in the quotes above, that one person can know what's best for someone else and *to act upon that opinion* when the power exists. In my opinion, these "benign" motives pose a great potential for abuse.

The most bothersome and likely abuse will come in the form of exterminating people who become "undesirable" to the government or another powerful group.

Compensating Piety

Most physicians will never be killers. They would be unable to accept themselves as a killer of even one innocent person, let alone a patient! Partly for this reason the armed forces do not require their medics to fight in combat. But physicians, motivated possibly by a sincere desire to ease suffering, may feel compelled to participate in "mercy killing" without fully considering the ramifications.

However, a physician's subconscious mind may continue to struggle with the contradiction in a way that threatens his or her sanity. Lacking an adequate resolution of their moral contradiction, some may seek to compensate their questionable behavior with completely dissociated unquestionable deeds. Dr. Robert Jay Lifton's study of the Nazi doctors describes how this split progresses: "[The Nazi doctor] invested his wife and children—and that part of himself bound to them—with a quality of absolute purity and goodness. And he clung to that purity and goodness with the special intensity of a man being consumed by evil."[4]

Lifton explains how goodness and evil can reside in the same personality by what he calls the psychological principle of doubling: the division of the self into two functioning wholes so that each part acts as an entire self.[5]

In this manner a physician could be both healer *and* killer at the same time. But as the activity of the killer part of him develops, so much tension builds in his psyche that he must balance out that evil and its resultant guilt with more activities that appear good. Thus an observable compensating piety often develops, "a pattern that recurs throughout this study: the immersion of themselves in 'medical science' as a means of avoiding awareness of, and guilt over, their participation in a murderous project."

Physicians are quite prone to doubling, as are all professionals, because they have done so much good and people have frequently showered them with compliments. They can cover a lot of evil with that "surplus of good."

But after a while the *healer-killer* almost imperceptibly evolves into a *killer-healer*. Now his healing is done, though largely unconsciously, in order to cover his killings instead of his killings being done, as he first expected, to round out his healing techniques. He who destroys others destroys himself. The destroyer is destroyed. As Jesus said, "With the measure you use, it will be measured to you" (Matt. 7:2).

Lifton offers as support of this change the true example of some "idealistic young Americans, working in a mental hospital as conscientious objectors to war and violence, [who] reached the point where they 'helped to kill' deteriorating mental patients. While their actions are hardly genocidal, these people of notably developed ethical sensitivity were led by their environment to collude in killing."[6]

The pressure of our environment as communicated through the opinions of our peers has a tremendous influence on us. So it makes a great deal of difference what we as a society condone as legal. Before abortion was legalized, most advocates emphasized the lesser-of-two-evils argument. Those advocates did not publically predict the wholesale application it now commands only a few years hence. But now the general public has been greatly desensitized.

Euthanasia Is Not "Good Medicine"

In making their proposal for the Humane and Dignified Death Act, the Hemlock Society falsely claims that "helping to die with dignity has become part of good medicine today."

But that's just not true. No place in America today accepts active euthanasia, let alone considers it the standard of "good medicine." Certainly some individual physicians advocate it, but this statement clearly misleads the public.

If the author meant that good medicine helps people "die with dignity"—meaning with the best of medical care and without needlessly prolonging the dying process—then that certainly is the accepted goal. But almost no one agrees that killing a patient enhances his or her dignity.

Similarly, the Hemlock Society's conclusion, "that the *best answer to this problem is physician aid-in-dying*," misleads the public. Why a physician? Because he would be the most merciful representative in society? Then why make him into a killer, which destroys his merciful nature?

As a Society, We Need More Than Medical Technicians

Technical expertise does not make a person a good physician. Dr. Alfred Blalock of Johns Hopkins Hospital used to say that he could take a good high school student into the laboratory and train him or her to be an excellent surgeon. But he was quick to add that he'd never let that person operate on a patient because good surgical *judgment* had not yet had time to develop.

It is popular today in many fields to seek "value neutral" approaches to society's problems. First of all, I question the validity of the term "value neutral." Most expressions I have seen are far from neutral. In fact, proponents soon prove to be quite hostile to anyone who advocates an assertive value system; that is, anyone who claims to know what is right and wrong or what *should* be done. But that's another subject. In terms of medicine, I'm convinced that we make a great mistake to discourage active judgments concerning what is ethically good and bad, because sooner or later the suppression of ethical judgment will result in the loss of good medical judgment and will ultimately harm the patient.

Ethical judgment supports medical judgment. As a practicing surgeon, I have committed myself to developing the best judgment possible. This would be impossible to accomplish without taking an objective look at my work. (There's a difference between striving to be objective and striving to be neutral.) And here's where part of the problem lies.

I must see an operation I have performed as if someone else had done it. In this way, I can ask questions about the whole conduct of the operation and the care of the patient that I could not deal with if I asked the emotionally loaded question, "What did *I* do?" When I can detach myself from what I've done, then I can approach the case as critically as if someone else had done it.

At this point, I can transcend that actual case and ask the important questions: "What could have been done differently? What information should have been researched that would have resulted in better decisions? What should have been done to achieve better results?" Each case must be evaluated on the basis of what actually did and didn't happen.

By developing surgical judgment, I can modify my behavior for the good of each future patient I operate on.

After taking the objective stance I can ask the emotionally loaded question, "What did *I* do?" Here I need to examine myself, how I practice medicine, and what kind of a person I am and am becoming. This, then, moves into the realm of an ethical judgment. This whole process *must* be fostered.

How can a society have good, moral, trustworthy physicians rather than bad, immoral, deceiving doctors if it does not continually encourage ethical development and judgment? Furthermore, does scientific technology have the ability to develop the ethics or morality of its creators? It does not solve the problem of what's good for the patient; for only the scientist and the technican, the human beings, can exercise goodness. And like the technology he creates, the human being gets the ability to be moral from his Creator. This happens regularly when the goodness of God flows *through* human hearts.

I believe that if the medical profession accepts a role in active euthanasia, as it has for abortion on demand, the whole medical establishment will suffer severely and eventually collapse. Why? For several reasons. There will be an immediate division in the medical profession that will cut to the core of what it means to be a physician, a nurse, any caretaker. This split will affect everything in the field of medicine, as well as every doctor and nurse, causing great suspicion between them.

In addition, the greater the pro-killing segment grows, the more momentous pressure will form that can force all but the most resolute healer to turn to killing. There are several books on this topic as it occurred in Germany, but I'd suggest that you only need to read Dr. Robert Lifton's book *The Nazi Doctors*. Further, as Dr. Lifton and Otto Rank point out: "Human beings kill in order to assert their own life power. To that tenet may now be added the image of curing a deadly disease, so that genocide may become an absolute form of killing in the name of healing."

When we consider that abortion on demand projects the image of curing a problem—elimination of the fetus—then active euthanasia produces the same image of curing a problem: elimination of terminally-ill patients.

Echoes of Hope

Furthermore, if euthanasia should become legalized, many doctors will be pressured to compromise, leave the profession, or will find it impossible to qualify to practice from the outset. But I have hope that no matter what happens, many doctors and medical professionals will maintain their resolve to be healers and not killers.

Such ethical resolve can be seen in those medical professionals who have not yielded to the pressure from state legislatures to participate in the killing of criminals who have received the death sentence. Currently 16 states provide for the death penalty by lethal injection, but since an injection is "medicine" and has to be done precisely if it is to be effective, some states have attempted to enlist the aid of the medical profession in administering it. A recent article in the *American Medical News* discusses this:

> The Illinois statute passed in 1983 calls for a medically trained person such as a medical technician to insert the intravenous catheter that supplies the lethal dosage. It notes that the execution must be conducted in the presence

of two physicians, one of whom must pronounce death. The procedure also states that a complete physical exam must be conducted before the execution date and that the drugs and dosages may be altered and administered in quantities determined by a "qualified health care person."

Many physicians argue that the mere presence of an MD at an execution gives the impression of moral sanction by the profession. "Participation in a execution in any manner would be an unethical practice," said Alfred Kiessel, MD, chairman of the board of the Illinois State Medical Society, adding that "participation" could range from ordering and prescribing the barbiturates to monitoring a prisoner during the course of the execution.

. . . Anticipating that nurses would be substituted for physicians who refuse to participate in lethal injections, the American Nursing Association's Committee on Ethics adopted its own policy in 1983. It states that nurses' participation either directly or indirectly in legally authorized executions would be a breech of the nursing code of professional ethics.[7]

I pray that as the issues become clearer, the same resolve will characterize my profession by its resisting any participation in or condoning of euthanasia.

Notes

[1] "Medical Ethics and the Issue of Torture," JAMA, Vol. 255, No. 20, May 23/30, 1986, p. 2798.
[2] Robert Jay Lifton, *The Nazi Doctors* (New York: Basic Books, 1986), p. 394.
[3] Howard Caplan, M.D., "It's Time We Helped Patients Die," *Medical Economics For Surgeons*, July 1987.
[4] Lifton, p. 396.
[5] Ibid., p. 418.
[6] Ibid., p. 498.
[7] Barbara Dow, *American Medical News*, September 4, 1987, pp. 9–10.

PART FOUR

Imparting Hope

CHAPTER TEN

On the Psychology of Dying

Much of the psychology of dying evolved subsequent to the development of life-support systems. As the ability of medical science to prolong life increased, the interval between life and death broadened and became a larger part of the human experience for both the dying person and his or her family, friends, relatives, and the medical staff, especially the nurses. This "living-dying interval" has been extended far beyond what many thought possible some years ago. And it will likely extend much further in the future.

So we have had the occasion to study death in much greater detail.

The Experience of Dying

The living-dying interval, says Dr. E. Mansell Pattison, professor of psychiatry at the Medical College of Georgia, begins with a crisis. From the moment of finding out the diagnosis that your condition is terminal until the moment you die comprises the living-dying interval. During this period, the patient goes through an acute crisis phase (1–2 in the diagram below) which finally peaks and then gradually declines until death. The chronic phase (2–3) ends in the final few days or weeks in the terminal phase (3–4).[1]

THE LIVING-DYING INTERVAL		
ACUTE PHASE	CHRONIC PHASE	TERMINAL PHASE
1————2———————————————————————3————————4		
Crisis of Peak		Rapid Final
Knowledge Anxiety		Decline Death

The Acute Phase

The news that a person has a terminal condition and will die in the relatively near future starts an anxiety reaction which builds constantly until it peaks at such a time that he can use his psychological mechanisms to reduce the anxiety and start to cope. If the person has a well-formed mental defense system, he will be able to integrate living into a helpful style of dying. However, the opposite holds true as well. If the person has ineffective defenses, he will not be able to bring his living style into alignment with his dying needs.

How can the news that a person is going to die produce such an acute crisis? H.J. Parad in 1965 described the reasons.

1. By definition the crisis is insolvable in the immediate future. It's a crisis to which we bow but do not solve.
2. The problem taxes one's psychological resources since it is beyond one's traditional problem-solving methods. "My death is like no one else's."
3. The situation is perceived as a threat or danger to the life goals of the person. "I haven't finished my life yet."
4. The emotional tension peaks and then falls off gradually as the patient mobilizes his or her coping resources.
5. The crisis awakens unresolved problems from both the near and distant past. The patient faces both the immedi-

ate dying process and the unresolved feelings from his own lifetime and its inevitable conflicts, which include things such as dependency, passivity, conceit, and identity.[2]

The Chronic Phase

The chronic phase of the living-dying interval contains a number of fears, according to Dr. Pattison, which, if the patient deals with them one at a time, can be resolved in a rewarding fashion. When meeting these fears adequately, the patient can experience strong feelings of self-control, self-esteem, and integrity. Throughout all of life few things give us as much dignity as struggling through a crisis. When we can cope successfully, we actually come out stronger and more mature.

I have personally cared for a number of patients who said, after a particularly difficult illness or injury, that while they would not ask for more tragedy in their lives, they wouldn't trade theirs for anything. One elderly woman said—after five years of cancer in every bone in her body, extensive arthritis, and poor blood supply to her feet—that she wouldn't want to trade those five years with cancer for any other five years of her life.

The fears often faced by a person in the chronic phase of the living-dying interval, says Dr. Pattison, can be categorized as follows:

1. Fear of the unknown.
- What life experiences will I not be able to have?
- What is my fate in the hereafter?
- What will happen to my body after death?
- What will happen to my survivors?
- How will my family and friends respond to my dying?
- What will happen to my life plans and projects?
- What changes will occur in my body?
- What will be my emotional reaction?
- Will I have excessive suffering? Can I handle it?

2. Fear of loneliness. Many aspects of dying produce loneliness for the patient.

- The sickness itself usually causes both patient and visitor to withdraw from each other.
- The delivery of medical care, especially by high-tech procedures, often places physical barriers between the patient and the caregivers.
- For the patient, the whole process of dying is isolating. He or she quits working, quits social activities, spends less time with hobbies, hasn't the strength to maintain daily activities with family, and his or her time becomes continually more consumed with caring for himself or herself than for others.
- Friends find it increasingly more difficult to arrange times to visit the patient; and when they do, he or she is less interested in them. Friends lose interest in visiting. So the patient loses more interest in them and his or her surroundings.

3. Fear of loss. The losses the patient sustains during the dying process invade his whole life: job, future plans, strength and abilities, financial reserves, the pleasure of relationships with family and dear friends, and sometimes the loss of some bodily functions.

4. Fear of losing family and friends. Many people feel too embarrassed to admit it, but the loss of close relationships causes a disaster until the terminal phase when the dying process itself leaves little room for thoughts of anything else. During the living-dying interval the patient often fears the reaction of their closest companions, their expression of sorrow and grief. Awareness of and gentle honest dealing with this fear brings much peace and joy.

5. Fear of loss of body. The progress of a terminal illness may require surgical, chemotherapeutic, and/or radiological treatment—all of which can result in gross changes of the body externally (such as loss of hair) and functions of the body internally. And each change signifies something of the certainty of the impending death, and possible rejection by others, even family members. And often such a change threatens self-esteem.

6. Fear of losing self-control. Dying means loss, loss of everything temporal. The process of dying, then, means a process of loss. The patient cannot be fooled. He or she knows whether anyone says it or not. The loss of strength and energy reaches a point which the patient has never experienced. "If I am not dying, why am I not getting well?" the patient thinks and often states aloud. As these functions diminish, the patient begins to suspect that he may lose more control of his bodily functions and mental abilities than he would like. And the fear of loss of self in increments can become crushing.

7. Fear of suffering and pain. This fear often cries loudest. A measure of pain when one feels strong is one thing, but when one has no energy to cope with it, it can be overwhelming. Suffering occurs when pain has no meaning, no explanation. Sometimes we see patients with pain that remains uncontrollable even with higher doses of medication than other people require for similar causes of pain. Pain obviously contains a very subjective side. However, evidence seems to indicate that tolerance to pain reponds largely to one's attitude. Severe, uncontrollable pain usually does not occur as an isolated event. Most often other fears or worries have not been resolved, and they contribute to the strength of the pain. When people have severe pain, it can so drain their energy that they are unable to care about anything else, not even life itself.

8. Fear of loss of identity. The fears described above all have something to do with loss of identity. Family, friends, job, home, and church each have an important part in sustaining our sense of identity in the present and past. Our plans, projects, and desires all create a sense of self in the future. The dying process, however, disrupts all of these moorings, and a person's sense of identity can suffer as a result.

But some things can compensate and stabilize one's sense of identity. They accomplish this by helping to maintain self-esteem, dignity, and integrity which reinforce the person's identity. Consider the following list:

- *Contact with others* who have been part of the person's life. As these people interact with the dying person, their human touch assures the patient that he or she is a unique person with as much worth as always.
- *The continuation of one's life* through one's children, life work, and the dispersal of one's possessions to others.
- *A desire for reunion with loved ones* who have died before or will die and join them later.

9. Fear of regression. The deterioration of the bodily functions causes an inevitable diminution of one's finest mental capacities. For some patients this means that they will behave in immature ways, sometimes unaware of their actions, but at other times embarrassingly conscious that their comments and attitudes and behaviors were inappropriate. Couple the mental immaturity with the loss of control of bodily functions and a person can regress into an almost infantile state which demands constant care.

While all people do not regress this much, many people fear this will happen to them. As the process of dying nears the terminal phase, the person continually loses interest in the world about him and is consumed increasingly with his own bodily problems and what it takes to live. Here the sense of time, space, or person disappears, leaving no boundaries between self and others.

The Terminal Phase

Finally the patient enters the terminal phase of dying. Usually the process of withdrawing into oneself begins this phase. The failing body demands more and more time and energy to remain alive until it takes more energy and work to live than to die. Weakening of the emotions can also occur and produce impatience, easy crying, lack of enthusiasm, and a depressed response even to human stimuli. The social cares and worries of daily life disappear, and finally the patient withdraws completely: dies.

Dr. Pattison mentions a change in hope as a sign that the terminal phase has begun. At first the patient has *expectational hope.* The expectation of not dying colors everything he or she says. But the terminal phase brings about the realization of the certainty of death. Then the patient switches to a *desirable hope.* Now he or she desires recovery but does not expect it anymore.

I have seen this in patients when they recognize for themselves that death *is* coming soon. From that point their attention centers on the dying process, and they begin making preparation for it. Instead of an attitude of "I'm going to get well," they slip into one of "It would be nice if I didn't die."

Most people arrive at this point unprepared for the actual experience of death. We may expect only sweetness and light as the dying person slips away with a few profound "last words." And by helping a person prepare for the moment of death, we do everything possible to make the passage smooth. But even the Bible acknowledges death as a cruel enemy, and we should not be surprised at the violent throes of death: a final struggle, a crying out for help rather than assuring words from the patient that they see Jesus inviting them to step into the realms of glory.

But a rough final round does not mean defeat. Our victory comes, after all, through the resurrection of Christ and not as a result of our personal performance.

The Meaning of Death

For many people death has no meaning, no significance except to end life completely. As a result they find themselves not only mourning their death but asking, "What good is life?" With Albert Camus they often conclude that life is the absurd lie, for life has no meaning.

Yet other people have found meaning in both life *and* death. Christian spokesman Francis A. Schaeffer wrote, "When we were created, we were created for a purpose. And the purpose of our creation, in which all our subsidiary purposes fit, is to be in a personal relationship to God, in communion with Him in love, by choice, the creature before the Creator."[3]

Only the human being, out of all earth's creatures, has been given the responsibility for developing into the creature he or she was created to be. I have seen some of my patients pursue this purpose even in the midst of great suffering.

Meaning Begins in Life

Why do some pursue personal development but not others? I found that those who continue to grow personally choose not to remain primarily interested in their bodies but go beyond the physical to the spiritual. They see their responsibility to become what God created them to be: spiritually centered beings, God's companions.

In *Escape From Evil*, Ernest Becker concluded, "To finish one's personality is to respond to faith which asks man to expand himself trustingly, to transcend himself in God and find meaning for his existence in God."[4]

Having faith in God did not come easily for most of the people I have attended during their final days. Yet after these patients worked through their doubt and fear, they found wholeness of personality in Jesus Christ.

We too need to struggle for faith in order to be sure that we truly desire to commune with God. How else can we be certain that we will enjoy living with God for eternity if we haven't experienced Him as our primary source of joy in this life? King David wrote a psalm about this: "But as for me, my contentment is not in wealth but in seeing You and knowing all is well between us. And when I awake in heaven, I will be fully satisfied, for then I will see You face to face" (Ps. 17:15, TLB).

Many people relate to God as they do to me—as a therapist whose role is to cure *their* ills. Often they have given time and money to God's causes. So when they suffer, they feel God should return the favor and help them.

Leslie D. Weatherhead was disturbed by this kind of attitude:

> I am often troubled by the querulous people who come to me in some distress or another and say, "I have prayed to God and I do trust God." "I've gone to church all my life . . . and I say my prayers night and morning."
>
> They have made no serious quest to get into that joyous relationship with God of the child to the loving father. They want God as they want anything—a tonic, or an operation, or any other kind of treatment would give them health or ease.[5]

Unless such people change their attitudes and give their sufferings to Christ, they will not be able to deal adequately with their pain. Ultimately my patients who are seeking and growing develop a steadfast faith, unshaken not only by the problems of life but by the inevitability of their own deaths.

The Anticipation of Immortality

In his excellent book *Voices of Death,* Edwin Shneidman, professor of thanatology at the UCLA School of Medicine, introduces the topic of meaninglessness with the following confession: "Marie Bashkirtseff, a well-to-do young Russian woman dying of tuberculosis in nineteenth-century Paris wrote, 'This is the thought that has always terrified me; to live, to be so filled with ambition, to suffer, to weep, to struggle, and, at the end, oblivion! as if I never existed.' "[6] The desire for immortality echoes from this cry for meaning. Why? Because the search for meaning always leads us to the inescapable conclusion of immortality, not just in symbols or within the confines of human survival as a race. But there must be a real life after death, which makes all that this life has to offer valuable and worthy of human endeavor.

When one denies the possibility of a real afterlife, the meaning and purpose of this earthly life is lost also. Albert Camus called this the absurd situation: "the confrontation between the human need and the unreasonable silence of the world."[7] In contrast to Camus, consider this statement by Robert N. Butter: "After one has lived a life of meaning, death may lose much of its terror. For what we fear most is not really death but a meaningless and absurd life." Indeed, Shneidman found "the desire for immortality seems to be one of the strongest drives in those who write about their dying."[8]

In the stark reality of life lies the fact that every person must die. No matter how we look at life, this fact continually awaits us and signifies the end of everything we do. If we deny this fact too much through our growing years, we will be unprepared to face it in our parents, family, friends, and in ourselves.

The Death Equivalents

In order to face our death without becoming overwhelmed, view the passages in this life as "death equivalents." In our society, for instance, graduation from high school marks the end of one's basic education and an acceptance as an adult. Once we graduate, we cannot return to that segment of our lives, even if we wanted to do so. Even to *visit* the high school, we are obliged to obtain official permission. So graduation symbolizes the end of an era, the death of being a minor and birth into adulthood.

For these experiences to be endings there must be some loss or grief that follows in their wake. Because of this, we can prepare for the deaths and griefs in our lives that must come. We are never able to replicate death by the practice run, but because of our smaller death equivalents, we can understand the reaction and the feelings that will be produced. Then we can work through the grief experience more fully since we won't be so overcome by the process itself.

Many times we go through difficult situations wondering, "Why is this happening to me?" Then, when time eases the pain and suffering, we forget about it, and we haven't applied it to the learning processes of life. But we could use the difficult transitions we face along the way to develop our ability to cope with our final passage from this life. We can learn that each contains a source of new life worthy of hope and anticipation. Each thread in the very woof and warp of life's fabric contains the pattern that teaches us to expect immortality.

Therefore, the *way* one dies almost always reflects the way one has lived through the darker times of life, the death equivalents. If a person does not experience any hope or value or opportunity in life's darker experiences, he or she will have a difficult time finding anything good in the dying process. At this point people tend to explore the idea of suicide—euthanasia.

Shneidman found that when a person who contemplates suicide finds meaning, their suicidal compulsion dissolves even though they may remain in great physical pain. In contrast he says, "The suicidal person is always in psychological pain, wishing to escape intolerable emotional distress."[9]

And how frequently we see this in dying patients! I recall an elderly woman on whom I had operated two years before to remove a cancer of her colon. On her second hospital admission we found a cancer in her pancreas and a return of more cancer in her colon. On operating, I discovered that these were too large to remove. During the ensuing weeks and months she suffered a lot. Finally one day she asked me about death. "How long will it take to die? I'm tired of suffering and fighting the pain," she confessed. "Do you believe in giving people something to put them to sleep permanently, if they want it?"

Her bodily pain and the excessive emotional turmoil clouded her perception of life. However, as this woman acknowledged her anxiety and insecurity, she began to see her dying as a part of her life. And as she reviewed her life and the many times she had come through other dark times, she decided not to give in to her disease, no matter what. She became an inspiration to me and her daughters.

Beyond Death's Door

What evidence do we have of life beyond the grave? To begin with, God has made our world in such a way that we have abundant opportunities to find Him. He has planted evidence throughout nature for us to see His sovereignty. Year after year, nature rehearses the themes of death and immortality through the seasons. Just as plants and trees seem to die in the dead of winter and then suddenly burst forth with new life and growth in the spring, so we can gain confidence that we too will live after our own winter of death.

Journalist Lincoln Barnett states in *The Universe and Dr. Einstein,* "In the evolution of scientific thought, one fact has become impressively clear: there is no mystery of the physical world which does not point to a mystery beyond itself."[10] Man's inescapable impasse, according to Barnett, is that he himself is part of the world he seeks to explore. Therefore, the only world we can truly know is the world created for us by our senses. Moreover, what we know outside our senses we have only representations of. We have to make some assumptions about those representations.

For instance, the planet Pluto—invisible to the naked eye—was first discovered in 1905 by the American astronomer Percival Lowell who calculated that the force of gravity of some unknown planet seemed to be affecting the orbits of Neptune and Uranus. From something he could observe, he made assumptions about something that he could not see, and he predicted the location of a new planet. Though he searched for years with a telescope, he died without ever seeing the planet. In fact, it was not until 1930 that a more powerful telescope photographed it right where he said it would be.

A Christian perspective, however, embraces more than evidences in our physical world that point to life beyond our senses. We have the Word of God, the Bible, and its recorded accounts of Jesus' raising people from the dead: a widow's son, a little girl, Lazarus. As our supreme example we point to Jesus' death and resurrection. He said, "I am the resurrection and the life. He who believes in Me will live, even though he dies; and whoever lives and believes in Me will never die" (John 11:25).

Death as Defeat? or Transition?

As Christians we can be certain that physical death does not end human existence. As many times as I have seen people die, I am reassured by Christ's resurrection that death is not the end of life. But an awareness of death can encourage us to make more of our lives now. So how can we find meaning in the fact of death?

Most of my patients begin by fearing death. When suffering strips people of their energies and abilities, they often wonder if they are about to die. They begin to question why they have lived, what value their life has been, and whether they have succeeded in becoming the person they were created to be. But that's OK; out of that questioning comes a strong motivation to reexamine their lives and reorder their priorities.

I have found that most patients—even believers—are not fully ready to die when they first face death. I don't mean that they don't qualify for heaven; I mean they haven't finished their earth work. The process of examining one's life, putting things into perspective, and making peace with things that have happened or not happened can be an important part of our life's work. Yet many people haven't ever deeply asked themselves: "Can I love and respect myself in view of the person I have been?" and "Who or what have I served and lived for?" As Paul Tournier says, "Underlying every decisive choice there is a prior, fundamental choice, a spiritual one, the choice of one's God: What is your God? your mother, your own self-interests, your instincts, your pleasure, reason, science, or Jesus Christ?"[11]

When we think about such questions we sharpen our self-image. Ernest Becker comments: "Man wants to know that his life has somehow counted, if not for himself, then at least in a larger scheme of things, that it has left a trace, a trace that has meaning. Or if there is to be a 'final tally of the scurrying of man on earth—a judgment day'—then this trace of one's life must enter that tally and put on record who one was and that what one did was significant."[12]

All of us want to tie the loose strings of life together and know that our lives have had purpose. Jesus Christ said we can find the highest meaning and purpose for life if we seek first the kingdom of God. (See Matthew 6:33.) Do we believe Him? God calls us to live holy lives. The Prophet Micah said, "What does the Lord require of you? To act justly and to love mercy and to walk humbly with your God" (Micah 6:8). Jesus Christ said that "whoever wants to save his life will lose it, but whoever loses his life for Me will find it" (Matt. 16:25).

Dignity in Death

At first glance, death seems to be the greatest indignity known to mankind. It is the only experience that humbles every human being and brings each of us to the end of our lives. Death is no respecter of persons. All have to die and none of us can decide for sure when that will be (unless we initiate death prematurely). Death deprives us of our greatest yearning: to live on and on and on.

As a physician, I rarely meet a person who thinks that the time of his or her death is appropriate. For instance, at 50 some think they'll be ready to die at 90. But that same person at 90 doesn't particularly want to die just then. I know several people in their 90s who would like to live several more years.

But if we call death the ultimate indignity, how can it sometimes be a great honor? For instance, when one person gives his life to save the life of another we attach no indignity. Jesus particularly spoke of this when He said, "Greater love has no one than this, that one lay down his life for his friends" (John

15:13). And then He demonstrated this by dying on the cross that we might have immortality.

Throughout the centuries those who gave their lives for others have been revered as being very dignified people. Dignity starts with the living process and is determined by the individual person, not what happens to him or her. Dignity therefore, comes from within a person rather than from without. No matter how hard others try to bestow "dignity" upon a person, this does not change the person's responsibility for his own dignity.

Viktor Frankl said it beautifully when he discussed the reactions of people in the concentration camps in Nazi Germany during World War II:

> Man is ultimately self-determining. What he becomes—within the limits of endowment and environment—he has made out of himself. In the concentration camps, for example, in this living laboratory and on this testing ground, we watched and witnessed some of our comrades behave like swine while others behaved like saints. Man has both potentials within himself; which one is actualized depends on decisions but not on conditions.[13]

The dignity of those people was determined by the individuals and not decided by the guards or the environment of the concentration camp.

So it is in our dying. There are numerous things external to us that appear to inhibit our expression of dignity: coma, paralysis, medication, senility, unbearable pain, isolation, insanity, ignorance, etc. Even our impersonal technological care via life-support systems can severely limit most expressions of human dignity, but not one's true dignity.

Finding Meaning in Suffering

The agony of dying frequently causes people to despair in the middle of the dying process itself. A number of my dying patients have said that they didn't fear death. What they did fear is the dying process. One man in particular phrased it this way: "I wouldn't mind death if I didn't have to go through the process." How often have you wanted to avoid the process of change, especially if you didn't ask for it? Yet change comes right down to the basics of life; struggling through the hard times brings new strength and growth—often new life. Jesus demonstrated on the cross that there is no life without death. He also spoke of the seed needing to die before new life begins.

In great American tradition we cheer for the underdog as he reaches deep into himself and finds the true grit needed to win. Our hearts are warmed and inspired when we see a handicapped person struggle through what seems an impossible situation and succeed. Every one of us has had the opportunity to go through a situation that we felt was impossible and undesireable. Yet when we persevered, we finally came through it better persons. Even the miracle of our salvation through Christ Jesus comes only after we are willing to die to self in order to be born anew in Christ.

And many of us have discovered that our greatest contribution to others has often come out of our own desperate experiences, after which we felt called to help others going through similar situations. Consider Charles Colson, Elizabeth Elliot, Helen Keller to suggest a few. A partial listing would take books to record.

The proponents of euthanasia state that terminal illness—particularly when laden with pain—is a meaningless experience and, therefore, euthanasia becomes the proper answer. And yet, as we have seen, despair and agony in the other transitions of life can have great purpose. Suffering is not necessarily valueless. What happens when we suffer can turn a trial into a triumph.

Finding the Best in the Worst

How can such a change occur? How can human beings, when faced with the worst, find the best? Specifically, how can a terminally ill person suffering from unbearable pain find meaning and hope in the dying process? The essence of the response can be seen in the preface to the English translation of *The Gulag Archipelago Three* by Alexander I. Solzhenitsyn: "The fighters' spiritual strength rises to the greatest height and to a supreme degree of tension when their situation is most helpless and the state system most ruthlessly destructive."[14]

Again we return to the cycle by which God matures us: life, death, and then life. However, it often occurs in softer, more elusive patterns, such as excitement, disappointment, excitement; advancement, setback, advancement; love, rejection, love; growth, decline, growth. But nowhere does the process of maturity become more important than in what I'd like to call our "life's masterpiece." Each person has a life to live, fashion, nurture, develop, and accomplish. The masterpiece: becoming the best person one can be. Our masterpiece begins as a small, precious gift from God, and it is our job to develop it to the fullest. In our daily living we discover this as the meaning and purpose of our lives.

The perception we have at any given moment can be greatly influenced, distorted, or inspired by the circumstances of life. Yet the true masterpiece consists of the inner quality of oneself through which self-worth and style of life may be comprehended.

Believing in God's Love for Us

Ten years ago while I was working on the topic of suffering and faith, I discovered that the essential character of faith is a struggle—a struggle to believe that God does truly love us and would never harm us. The same question arises in the process of death: Can we learn to trust Him enough in life to have confidence in Him for eternity and for the transition between the two?

I found that merely coping with problems and tragedies is not enough. We need to go beyond any trial by using it for growth and development. Growth depends on our willingness to struggle.

Our natural inclination is to interpret life's cycles as follows: health means God loves me; tragedy indicates God doesn't love me; then God expresses His love toward me, and I return to health. It takes our concerted exercise of faith to reach beyond a Pavlovian interpretation of life and believe that God loves us through ease or pain.

The same process of developing our faith occurs in regard to hope. This process could look this way:

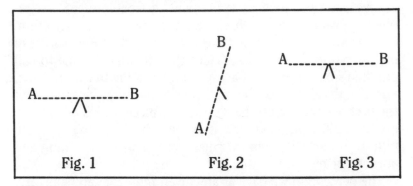

Fig. 1   Fig. 2   Fig. 3

Figure 1 shows a person in a comfortable balance with life. Figure 2 describes the imbalance in which the person stays at the bottom and the circumstance overwhelms him or her. But in figure 3 the person has overcome the problem and balance has returned—but more, the person now has matured to a level above the former plane. When another adversity occurs, the balance dips again for the person; then when he or she responds and grows, he or she attains a higher level balance.[15]

When a person is caught in the lower position of the tension—figure 2—he or she is easily discouraged and often loses perspective on the situation. A feeling arises that what was hoped for will never happen, that all the contents of life are lost. But it is at this specific point of deepest anxiety over the impossibility of the masterpiece of one's life ever occurring that one begins to see a far-off vague outline of hope. It's as if one could see oneself at the other extreme of the situation.

The Gift of Hope

As Solzhenitsyn found in the gulag, when a person's life situation is most hopeless and unending, then he is given hope that life is real and meaningful. Author Ira Progoff describes this event:

> Then with all the depths of his being he could believe in life. Hope was given to him, and it was a hope addressed to the full potentiality of life becoming manifest in all the forms of human existence. It was in this sense that the Psalmist could say, "My hope is in the Lord." The hope he placed in the Lord did not set restrictions on what God should do. The Psalmist did not specify what he hoped for. He simply affirmed his faith in the power of life and in its abundance. When hope is experienced as an unconditional affirmation of life there is an open relation to the unfolding possibilities of existence.[16]

All of us encounter circumstances which are so extreme that they go beyond the experiences of our past. When this happens that situation breaks the connection we have with our acquired resources and tests our ability to respond creatively. We are bankrupt, empty, broken. We feel as far removed from life as possible, alone, and—as it were—without a past or a future. The feeling of insignificance becomes so great that one cries out: "Is there anyone who can help me?"

Then, at first almost imperceptibly, but later, if we pursue it more strongly through prayer, comes the positive response of God Himself. He gives the hope of life with His unlimited resources. This hope comes from God and centers in Him, the Author and Creator of life. And then the broken connection with life is reestablished and the whole of life becomes a possibility.

Progoff studied Leo Tolstoy's writing *My Confession,* in which Tolstoy asked himself what the meaning of his life was. Progoff found that in the depths of despair Tolstoy wrote:

"I began to pray to Him whom I sought that He would help me. But the more I prayed, the clearer it became that I was not heard, that there was no one to whom one could turn." And later, "Lord, have mercy on me and save! O Lord, my God, teach me!" And finally, "I cannot help seeing that someone who loved me brought me into being. Who is that someone? Again the same answer—God. He knows and sees my search, my despair, my struggle. 'He is,' I said to myself. I had only to admit that for an instant to feel the possibility of existing and the joy of it."[17]

I have seen many terminally ill patients have this experience. Dying can bring a patient to the point of despair, concluding that life has no meaning, and making him or her feel lost, alone, and insignificant. The prospect of one's own death and the way pain and disease can sap one's energy can overwhelm the dying person. Often at this point the patient turns his interest more to dying than living. Many will ask about something that will hurry up the process.

But we can make a big mistake by answering this question in the affirmative because this moment forms part of the process of inner growth and experience with life. As we have seen from the above description of the dynamic tension between anxiety and hope, this point of despair occurs as a natural process with a built-in, inherent answer. So our task remains to support the dying person while he or she finds hope and meaning in life and death.

A Case in Point

I recall a woman who entered her terminal phase when cancer spread to her lungs. She became so weak and short of breath that she could only say a word or two at a time. One day when I went into her hospital room she was crying. She said that she had become a worthless person and a burden to everyone. She could see no meaning in her suffering and thought that she could do nothing significant for anyone else.

I told her that she was worthwhile and that's why I was spending so much time caring for her. I asked her to describe her dying process when she could. She stayed mentally alert and closer to God in that regard than I or any of the people who came regularly to help her. I asked her to think about that and share her experience with us.

Over the next few days I noticed little change. Then one day I immediately saw her smile as I approached her bed. She said, "I've been sharing." She had told a number of people what her new relationship with God was like. Through this new vision of God she regained her self-worth and found even her dying process meaningful.

Notes

[1] E. Mansell Pattison, *Experience of Dying* (Englewood Cliffs, New Jersey: Prentice Hall, Inc., 1977), pp. 48–55.

[2] H.J. Parad, ed., *Crisis Intervention: Selected Readings* (New York: Family Service Association of America, 1965).

[3] Francis A. Schaeffer, *True Spirituality* (Wheaton, Illinois: Tyndale House, 1971), p. 88.

[4] Ernest Becker, *Escape From Evil* (New York: The Free Press, 1975), p. xvii.

[5] Leslie D. Weatherhead, *Why Do Men Suffer?* (New York: Abingdon, 1936), p. 209.

[6] Edwin Shneidman, *Voices of Death* (New York: Harper & Row, Publishers, 1980), p. 5.

[7] James W. Woelfel, *Camus: A Theological Perspective* (Nashville: Abingdon Press, 1975), p. 44–45.

[8] Shneidman, p. 5.

[9] Ibid., p. 54

[10] Lincoln Barnett, *The Universe and Dr. Einstein* (New York: The New American Library of World Literature, 1952), p. 127.

[11] Paul Tournier, *The Meaning of Persons* (New York: Harper & Row, 1957), p. 209.

[12] Becker, p. 4.

[13] Viktor E. Frankl, *Man's Search for Meaning,* (New York: Washington Square Press, Inc., 1963), p. 213.

[14] Alexander I. Solzhenitsyn, *The Gulag Archipelago Three* (New York: Perennial Library, Harper & Row, Publishers, 1979), p. xi.

[15] The best description I have found of this development of hope comes from Ira Progoff in his book *The Dynamics of Hope* (New York: Dialogue House Library, 1985).

[16] Ibid., p. 82.
[17] Ibid., p. 54.

CHAPTER ELEVEN

How To Provide Comfort and Compassion

As we have noted, the use of our new technology reduces the human contact between doctor and patient. For the physician the new technology means a higher level of scientific care, the survival of a number of patients who would otherwise die, and the extended care of many more. Yet all this favoritism for high tech has left the patient lonely, isolated, and often depressed. Certainly the major roles of the medical profession have not actually changed in theory but in practice.

Learning to Care

When the human interface slowly diminishes, so does the compassion, comfort, and trust which normally occurs when two humans respond to each other in warm communion.

But as Christians, our primary way to care for dying persons must come expressly through a concerted effort to maintain contact. Why through contact? Because the basis of what we have to give lies in the relationship we have with them. Our basis for caring for others arises from God's care for us. Jesus did not have to die for us. He could have called resources from heaven and defeated the human mob that nailed Him to the cross, but He did not.

Jesus died on the cross because He wanted to accomplish

our redemption. By enduring the cross—the worst type of death—He showed us that He wanted to not only empathize with us, but He wanted to join us in *our* sorrow.

The Source of Compassion

Jesus enters into our suffering, supports us, gets under the load with us and actually helps us carry it. He suffers with us. He proved this in His life on earth. He cried, wept, was moved with compassion—whatever was necessary to identify with those who suffered. In so doing He lightened their load and led them through their misery to a higher plane of living beyond their grief.

This does not mean that He takes our suffering away from us and makes life simple. But He takes each situation and helps prepare us for the next higher level.

This was clearly true with Corrie ten Boom when she was dying after several strokes and could not talk or communicate. (See her story in Chapter 13.) People who came to see her and comfort her were remarkably aware of the presence of God in Corrie's room. He was there going through Corrie's dying with her and leading her to eternity. He did not suddenly take Corrie's place in the dying bed and send Corrie off on a holiday until He died for her. But He went through her dying with her.

It is quite significant that before Jesus returned to heaven, he said He would send the "comforter"—or in Greek, the *parakletos,* or one who comes alongside to help us.

How *We* "Come Alongside" Others

Each of us who has the Spirit of Christ abiding in us can take the Lord into every situation where another person suffers and share Him with that person.

This does not mean that we whip up a compassion for the terminally ill through our own power. On the contrary, it means that we share with others the very same compassion and comfort that we have received from God.

The Apostle Paul explains this in detail:

> Praise be to the God and Father of our Lord Jesus Christ, the Father of compassion and the God of all comfort, who comforts us in all our troubles, so that we can comfort those in any trouble with the comfort we ourselves have received from God. For just as the sufferings of Christ flow over into our lives, so also through Christ our comfort overflows. If we are distressed, it is for your comfort and salvation; if we are comforted, it is for your comfort, which produces in you patient endurance of the same sufferings we suffer. And our hope for you is firm, because we know that just as you share in our sufferings, so also you share in our comfort (2 Cor. 1:3-7).

What a relief to know that the Lord will pass on through us the compassion and comfort that others need. This frees us from a load of anxiety wondering how we should comfort others. Before we visit, we will be inspired and encouraged by spending time with God recounting both His compassion for us and the comfort He has given so abundantly in our problems and trials.

Recall the many sufferings and trials that Paul endured after his conversion and decision to follow Christ. It is this man who tells us of the praise and promise of God: "Praise be to the God . . . who comforts us in all our troubles, so that we can comfort those in any trouble with the comfort we ourselves have received from God."

From this perspective we can understand how all our problems and trials can become a source of mutual experience with those whom we wish to comfort. We have great confidence in God and His ability to comfort others because we have experienced His faithfulness to us. Just as Paul could say to the Corinthians, "For just as the sufferings of Christ flow over into our lives, so also through Christ our comfort overflows," so we can share with confidence the comfort of Christ. Remember that the Spirit of Christ Himself stands as the mediator between us and the patient. We are not left alone with the patient. Our fellowship with others flows through the Spirit who connects our spirit with the spirit of the patient.

Lloyd J. Ogilvie says, "It's in our relationships that we are the Good News we seek to share."[1] The actual relationship you have with another person communicates the Gospel more than what you say. If the hurting person finds peace in his relationship with you, then he has experienced something of the peaceful relationship available with God.

A paraphrase of Albert Schweitzer will clarify this point: "And through those whom He indwells, whether they be simple or wise, He will reveal Himself in the relationships they have, in the fellowship with the suffering and hurting people they serve. And as an ineffable mystery those served shall see the image of God in His servants."

The Avenues of Compassion

By what power or dynamic can we achieve such a wonderful relationship with people? Simply by the presence of the Spirit of Christ in us. Paul explained it this way: "But the fruit of the Spirit is love, joy, peace, patience, kindness, goodness, faithfulness, gentleness, and self-control. Against such things there is no law. . . . Since we live by the Spirit, let us keep in step with the Spirit" (Gal. 5:22-25).

As we work with others and particularly the hurting ones, let us concentrate on this fruit asking God to help us share the fruit that the patient needs the most. God will be faithful! As you experience God working through you, your soul will be thrilled and fulfilled. Indeed, you will be a *joyful comforter* as you comfort others.

The Extent of Compassion

Is there a situation too severe for this kind of spiritual comfort? Paul says NO!

We do not want you to be uninformed, brothers, about the hardships we suffered in the province of Asia. We were under great pressure, far beyond our ability to endure, so that we despaired even of life. Indeed, in our hearts we felt the sentence of death. But this happened that we might not rely on ourselves but on God, who raises the dead. He has delivered us from such a deadly peril, and He will deliver us. On Him we have set our hope that He will continue to deliver us (2 Cor. 1:8-10).

What a statement of God's great depth of compassion and comfort! Even when Paul despairs so much that he'd rather die than go on suffering (have euthanasia?), God has a better plan. When Paul quit trying to solve his own agonizing condition, God himself comforted Paul far beyond any human possibility. Yes, I wholeheartedly agree, for I've witnessed this in a number of my patients, as well as in my own life. When human resources are bankrupt, God supplies our deepest needs.

The Practice of Compassion

But how can we as human beings develop the attitudes that will allow the compassion and comfort God gives to flow through us?

1. Relate to others as full-fledged human beings of personal worth. As Jesus said, "Love your neighbor as yourself." They have been created by God, people for whom Christ died in order that they might be reconciled to God. In addition we are ambassadors: "God making His appeal through us." It is not so much what we do or say but the persons we are.

2. Dynamic listening. Our goal in assisting hurting people lies in helping them carry their burdens. Often when a hurting person talks they speak out of their pain which has been enclosed in layers of emotion. Therefore, we need to help them penetrate through their emotions in order to get to the real issue. Such camouflaged communication is sometimes called "encoded messages."

The aim of dynamic listening, then, centers on helping to decode the message. Decoding remarks sound like this: "Tell me more about that." "Explain how that happened." "I might have misunderstood, but were you saying . . . ?" "I get the feeling that you're really . . . (upset, angry, mad, frustrated, or whatever the emotional tone you pick up). Go on. I want to hear what you are saying." "How do you feel about it?"

All of these responses to the patient are designed to encourage the person to explore his or her own feelings and perception. Dynamic listening, therefore, encourages patients to talk about whatever they want. The patient leads the conversation and indicates by words, lack of words, and body language what type of response he or she would like at any given time.

Sometimes patients want us only to be sounding boards for their feelings. Dynamic listening does more than talking. Sometimes the dynamic requires silence, crying, holding a hand, or even giving a hug. By dynamic listening the visitor listens to the patient's whole personality and then responds in helpful ways.

Asking questions and urging someone to answer has its place, but it isn't always the most helpful way to listen. The anticipation of death often includes the characteristics of grief, and well it should. The dying person will be losing much too. The late Joseph Bayly, who himself experienced great grief at the deaths of three of his children, said:

Sensitivity in the presence of grief should usually make us more silent, more listening. . . .

I was sitting, torn by grief. Someone came and talked to me of God's dealings, of why it happened, of hope beyond the grave. He talked constantly, he said things I knew were true.

I was unmoved, except to wish he'd go away. He finally did.

Another came and sat beside me. He didn't talk. He didn't ask leading questions. He just sat beside me for an hour and more, listened when I said something, answered briefly, prayed simply, left.

I was moved. I was comforted. I hated to see him go.[2]

3. Trust people to solve their own problems. Such trust is quickly noticed, and builds a person's self-esteem and confidence. By helping people make choices and take responsibility for themselves you help them control their dying process rather than be overwhelmed by it.

This brings us back to the question of dignity and personal identity, for our dignity and identity arise from within us as we make choices and take responsibility for the attitudes and responses we make to the circumstances that life gives us.

I cannot express strongly enough the importance of dynamic listening. With all of our high-tech medical care, the emphasis on treatment does not encourage dignity and clarity of personal identity. In fact, Dr. Melvin Krant points out:

> During the time in the hospital or nursing home, little effort is made to help a patient maintain any control of his environment. For the patient who must regress and give up self-control and responsibility in illness, the institution both supports and promotes further regression. As a part of the regressed behavior, consideration of a patient's rights and the need to openly discuss the meaning of his illness and of his potential dying are frequently ignored. Patients often come to respect the fact that there are few if any people in their environments with whom they can safely discuss the deep tensions within.[3]

Filling the Vacuum

What must the dying person really fulfill through his or her relationship with us?

Since we actualize the fullness of our personalities primarily in relationship with other people, the diminished contact dying patients have with other human beings greatly handicaps the last stages of a person's maturity on earth. Consequently, the patient often experiences a personal identity crisis. The perceived loss of identity worsens as the patient loses control of his environment, and later even his own bodily functions.

Reinforcing a Sense of Self

Dr. Shneidman points out the following principles, goals, and beliefs that have guided him as he has tried to reinforce the identity of dying persons:[4]

1. *The goal of increased psychological comfort.* The main goal of working with the dying person—in the visit, the give-and-take of talk, the advice, the interpretations, the listening—is to increase that individual's psychological comfort.
2. *The autonomy of the individual.* This idea is based on respect for the individual. The opportunity to control one's own treatment, to maintain a sense of dignity, and to be as free as possible of unnecessary pain should not be snatched from a person simply because he or she is dying.
3. *The pitfalls of transference.* People have a built-in proclivity for quickly transferring their rather important feelings to another person. One day as I was making rounds I entered the room of a terminally ill patient, and his wife spoke out and said, "I'm sure glad to see you this morning. Bill likes you and listens to whatever you tell him." That's all very nice if that's what Bill really wanted to tell me, but if his wife spoke presumptuously, it created a very awkward situation: does he acquiesce, deny the claim, or quietly demonstrate its untruth by deliberately not doing what I tell him?
4. *The goals are limited.* The therapist or helper needs to be able to tolerate incompleteness and lack of closure. No one ever untangles all the varied skeins of one's interpersonal life; to the last second there are interactions that require new resolutions. Total insight is

only theoretical. The emphasis is on the relationship and on the helper's continued presence. Nothing has to be accomplished.

So caring for the patient doesn't rest on a schedule. Listen, and he or she will lead the way. We can help clarify some of their feelings. This requires that we hear what they are saying. God gave us *two* ears and *one* mouth; that should tell us something! We should listen, ask if what we heard is what they want us to hear, and then listen again. The key is listening and helping them tell their own story better. We should have no agenda, nothing that we must get patients to say and no specific stages that they must go through. We do not visit for our sakes, but theirs.

Building Trust

Basic to the feeling of a need to control one's own life lies trust. This trust must include a belief and confidence—a conviction—that the caretakers will accept the patient as a full human being with dignity and personal worth. This trust provides the patient with a sense of control as the caretakers assume custody and guardianship of him. Without this level of trust a patient may become suspicious not only of the correctness of care but, more importantly, of his or her human dignity.

One of the most critical issues in building and maintaining trust for the patient is honesty—honesty about his medical condition. According to Dr. Thomas P. Hackett, chief of psychiatric consultation service at Massachusetts General Hospital in Boston, those people who are told the truth have fewer medical, emotional, and psychiatric complications than those from whom the truth has been withheld.[5] Psychologist Herman Feifel, in a California research project, discovered that 90 percent of terminally ill patients were in favor of being told their condition directly.[6] It is the patient's right to know and essential for maintaining trust.

Having suffered a diminution in human dignity, the patient faces a personal crisis in which the ordinary fears of illness, the unknown, and the controlling machines can become overwhelming. Therefore, as Dr. Melvin J. Krant, professor of psychiatry at Harvard, has taught:

> We must look at ways that help an individual feel in control of himself and feel safe in passing through fearful portals. It means a trust in the innate strength of most people to confront this area of human crisis in illness and dying, and help them to be a participant in decisions which affect the manner of their living and the style of their dying.[7]

Whether the patient desires a life-support system or not, the need to work through the dying process remains basic to the care of the terminally ill. Primarily we need to support their personal dignity with open discussion of how they want to handle their condition, how to confront the issue of death itself, and the roles of each person involved.

Thus trust between the patient, the health team, and the family provides a warmhearted personal network that provides the feeling of safety that the patient so desperately needs. But surrounded by machines, alarms, tubing, and monitors, patients infrequently receive that human touch in the modern high-tech hospital. So they have to manage their struggle for personal identity, self-esteem, and finding meaning in their living and dying in isolation. "The cold fact is," found Shneidman, "that most people die too soon, with loose threads and fragments of life's agenda uncompleted."

Repairing Bridges

A few years ago I had a young father who was dying of cancer of the lung as a patient. When he was hospitalized for the final time, he called every member of his immediate family into the room and made peace with them. Then he telephoned all his relatives, many in different states, and asked for forgiveness where necessary and restored their friendship. He said he shouldn't die with his life so upset.

But usually if a patient is going to address his final earth work, we will need to assist him or her in doing it. It is not good enough for us to expect the patient to ask for help or do a correct job alone. The truth of the old saying, "When a person is ready to die, he or she is ready to live," certainly can be seen at this point of family support. For the psychological and emotional problems of death arise not so much from the process of dying as from the unresolved problems of living.

For the family, it is often the impending death of a family member that confronts them with unsettled conflicts and damaging attitudes that need resolving.

Death signifies the end of relationships. Its approach calls for us to decide about the quality of those intimate family connections. Disturbing questions may awaken deep-seated anxieties in the whole family: Will we be satisfied after our loved one dies with our part of the relationship? Could we have been more understanding and forgiving, trusting and kind, peaceful and joyful? Should I have shared more of myself, my feelings, my thoughts, my concerns, and my delights about our relationship? Why did I deny it when we did not relate well? Why was I so protective and fearful of exposing him or her to the hard spots of life? Why did I try to keep the worst problems a secret? And now in the final days how can I say, "I love you; you can trust me"? How can I let her be in control of her dying when I controlled her living?

"The family that is open and supportive in helping a loved one to live with a fatal illness," writes Dr. Krant, "can be a great asset in helping a person to die well. When open communication between a person and his family has developed, with secrecy and collusion avoided, great strength for all exists." After family members work through their unresolved problems of living together and can face their loved one's death in constructive, helpful relationships, then they are not only prepared for death but ready to live.

This working-through process gives excellent preparation

for the patient in facing his or her own death since the key relationships of life form a vital part of life's masterpiece for every person. And this process effectively helps accomplish just what the dying family member wants. For one of the greatest meanings that we can find in our whole life comes specifically at this point of using our final months, and perhaps years, as an experience which in itself will enable one's loved ones to live and die well.

Helping Others Prepare

Helping others prepare for their own deaths can give dying persons an important purpose in their remaining days. Dying people receive so much from the care others give them that they gain self-worth by using their dying experience to prepare others for their own.

One of my patients who was dying of cancer of the breast commented several times that if going through the process of dying helps her family members with theirs, she would count it a worthwhile experience. And a number of my patients have told me that if they could teach me more about dying so that I could help others, they would feel that their dying process was valuable.

Tying It All Together

Many of us envision coming to our final phase of life hoping for a reprieve from the death sentence. However, our deeper hope centers on living and dying well. None of us wants to die having done an inadequate job of living our lives. And certainly no one wants to botch the drama of his or her life in its final act. Professor Shneidman sums up his book *The Voices of Death*, speaking to this point: "My fervent hope is that in the real performance of it [the drama of my own death], I won't act too badly. I do deeply desire that the 'reviews' of my dying won't speak too harshly on my way of having done it. It's a point of pride with me."[8]

The tragedy of euthanasia surfaces at this very point. It deprives the patient of the opportunity to put his or her whole life's work into practice during the final act of living. As E. Stanley Jones, a great world missionary, proclaimed, "Now I must apply what I have been preaching through the years: That no matter what happens to us, the final result depends on how we take it. Here I was to be called upon to illustrate and apply the Good News, the Divine Yes, in the face of the bad news life often offers."[9]

Dr. Jones' final book, *The Divine Yes,* was written during the final 14 months of his life during which he suffered from the physical handicaps of a major stroke, which had produced dehumanizing limitations on him. He was not able to preach, and his eyesight was so poor that he couldn't see his own handwriting. He could only dictate into a tape recorder. So his daughter and her husband used his recordings to write *The Divine Yes* for him. This book signified a culmination to his life. It brought who he was living for, Jesus Christ, into clear focus as the central theme of his life's masterpiece. It also gave his children a project by which they could work together on helping Dr. Jones live to the fullest during his final earth work.

The true life-support system for any human being, therefore, cannot be found in technology but in dynamic human relationships in which the patient as person is addressed and his personal needs are met. A patient's medical problems need to be treated with the best scientific care possible, but he or she also requires psychospiritual support.

Creating a Legacy

The essence of accepting death as a natural part of life centers in the opportunity that we have to improve the dying person's remaining life. One way we can do this is by reviewing the patient's life with him or her. To explore the patient's life, to see in it the production of a personality with many facets, and then to watch a central theme emerge, to observe the coming together of various themes and fragments, to review the contributions of that person to others, and especially to encounter God working through one's life—all this brings meaning to life and helps create a legacy of which one can be proud, that cannot be destroyed by pain and suffering.

If the dying person remains coherent and able to talk, here are a few suggestions for how friends and family members can help do this.

- Have the patient work with a family member on filling out a family tree.
- Using a tape recorder, get stories of ancestors that only he or she knew well.
- When grandchildren visit, have the dying person describe what his or her life was like at the age of the grandchildren. Help make the questions specific: "How did you get to school?" "What was your first job?"
- Offer help in dispersing small personal items (those not listed in a will) to those who would appreciate them.
- Ask what is the most important thing the patient has learned during his life. Would he want it shared with others—in a letter, at his funeral, etc.?
- Encourage the person to have some input in the planning of his or her funeral: What songs would they like to have sung? What Scripture do they want read? Whom would they like to speak?

As you support and encourage the patient in this final stage of his or her life's work, you will find yourself enriched and encouraged, as one generation passes on its legacy to another. And isn't this the final gift of a meaningful relationship? Even though a person may die, his or her life's masterpiece continues on to strengthen others as they face the challenges life brings, even that final challenge: facing death in a dignified and meaningful way.

Notes

[1] Lloyd J. Ogilvie, *Let God Love You* (Waco, Texas: Word Books, 1974), p. 13.

[2] Joseph Bayly, *The Last Thing We Talk About* (Elgin, Illinois: David C. Cook Publishing Co., 1969), pp. 55–56.

[3] Melvin J. Krant, *Dying and Dignity* (Springfield, Illinois: Charles C. Thomas Publisher, 1974), pp. 58–59.

[4] Edwin Shneidman, *Voices of Death* (New York: Harper & Row, Publishers, 1980), pp. 114–121.

[5] Bayly, p. 37.

[6] Ibid, p. 38.

[7] Krant, p. 81.

[8] Shneidman, p. 192.

[9] E. Stanley Jones, *The Divine Yes* (Nashville: Abingdon Press, 1975), back cover.

CHAPTER TWELVE

Preparing for Death as a Family

When I was a premed student at Purdue in the late 1950s, ICUs were relatively unknown. People died at home much more often than in the hospital. Very few tubes or machines cluttered the patient's room. A few intimate family members took care of the patient. And when the rest of the family and friends visited, they saw the dying person much the same as they had always known him, except for being in bed.

In today's ICU, one seldom finds the person they expect to visit. What stands out are the tubes, machines, monitors, and the hurry and scurry of nurses, technicians, doctors, and aides obscuring the patient. None of the visitors can draw close enough to the patient in the usual five minutes allowed to reassure the patient that they are there and really care. Instead, families gather in nearby waiting rooms for hours between visits and the patient frequently doesn't ever know that his loved ones have spent the whole day waiting in the hospital.

Furthermore television at least weekly displays these ICU scenes to millions of viewers but rarely emphasizes the patient-family relationship. Everything else, including the love life of the doctor, highlights the drama of dying. And we wonder why people see dying as a lonely, isolated process. And if the patient is featured, it is always to express the battle to overcome unbearable agony and rarely to demonstrate how much the life-support system helps the patient. Consequently, many people today have this picture in mind when they think of dying and conclude that the process of dying will be a tremendous burden on family and society.

"But I Don't Want to Be a Burden"

Our technologically advancing society considers old things worthless and a burden to have to use. The emphasis is on what's new. Progress means action. Without constant innovation, companies can even lose their competitive edge.

In computer software data bases, the leading giant for years has been AstonTate with Dbase. Even though it has been updated several times, it has been over two years since the current version, Dbase III Plus, was introduced. Consequently, AstonTate's chairman, Ed Esber, acknowledged: "We have been a little slow. We don't intend for that to happen again. We got a little lax, but to go from 100,000 lines of code to 400,000 is a big leap."[1]

Anything not new or that takes time loses its value very rapidly. In this atmosphere, no wonder so many old people are terrified by the prospect that they might some day become a burden on someone. And yet the very technology that forces us to keep up-to-date has also produced the life-support systems that have prolonged thousands of lives and also prolonged death for thousands of others. In this mode of thought sickness and dying are totally useless and damaging to the patient. Yet the societal emphasis of "the newer the better" remains in place.

The elderly that are not quite as sick are assigned to "out of the way" institutions until they die. In 1987 America's expenditure for long-term care services reached $36 billion. One projection indicated that of the 600,000 elderly people to be admitted to nursing homes in 1988, some 20 percent of them will spend more than $50,000.[2]

Add to this the weakening effects of chronic illnesses and the prospect of slow dying which largely constrict a person's ability to do anything constructive for the family or society (in a society where "doing" demonstrates worth), and it's no wonder that many elderly people find it hard to justify the time, energy, or money given for them to live until they die.

Some Families Don't Want to Be Bothered

Furthermore, an elderly parent doesn't want to "get in the way" of the children's family interaction and satisfying the needs of grandchildren. Frankly, most elderly parents do not feel that they are a part of their children's families. And they certainly don't want to compete with grandchildren for affection, time, or money.

Many families have forgotten their responsibility for grandparents. We live as if the old generation does not exist. As soon as our parents lose their independence—for whatever reason—they become a burden. Have someone else care for them. We want to be free to go on living the way we are, accumulating material things, traveling when and where we want to go. And when they do stay at home, we want peace and quiet without hassle. Many conclude that they have worked hard for what they have and deserve to enjoy it alone. "Besides," they say, "my parents don't understand the computer I have, they complain that my beautiful stereo music is too loud, and they usually have to have things a certain way or they get upset. It's such a bother!"

Older People Notice

This attitude of avoiding "bother" infects everything we do with the dependent elderly. No wonder they feel that they are burdens. Dr. Melvin Krant says:

The attitude of the others, those depended on, becomes

most important. People are suspicious of the unknown and frequently possess barriers and defenses against letting others come to know them. When such suspicion is fortified by an attitude of not caring to know in the caregivers, the sick are forced to turn inward into their loneliness and fears. Existing problems such as weakness, pain, breathlessness, or nausea become aggravated and exacerbated through fear, uncertainty, distrust, and loneliness. If one is uncertain as to who can be depended upon to truly help, an individual becomes even more alone in his suffering.[3]

Choosing an Alternative

In spite of these sad trends in our society, many of us don't want to "dispose of" old or infirm people. We value and love them and want to be with them through their approaching death. But how can we prepare our families for this? How can we be ready to stand by our loved ones? How can we help each family member become ready for his or her own death?

Preparation for death can begin by using the experiences of everyday life to illustrate basic concepts about death. Also, the dying experience of a family member itself can be used to prepare the remaining family for each other's deaths and for their own as well.

Let Death Speak

Whenever we attend to the dying we must—and this comes automatically, if we allow it—look at our own death. Until I've admitted my own mortality, have faced its implications for my life, and have begun to work through it, I cannot assist another person in his or her dying very much. What the dying person experiences brings about a response in me. And so I am forced to react within myself. And while this process goes on within me, I am so preoccupied with my own reactions that I'm not very available to hear the needs and concerns of the dying person. But once I have been able to face my own death and respond to it, I become much more sensitive to the needs of others.

Believe me. In my own experience I found a tremendous improvement in my ability to assist a dying person *after* I faced my own death. And it's not hard to tell which caretaker has worked through his or her death either.

Value *Being*

Why should facing one's death make such a difference? When we consider our own death deeply, we become enlightened by the difference between *being* and *doing,* and our appreciation for the *being* of the dying patient grows rapidly. So much of our existence in this life focuses on what one does, how much one accomplishes, what one might attain. When death looms close, a person's achievements pale, and we see more rightly the significance of what it is that God has created: a human being.

Our concern then takes a quick turn in the direction of nurturing that "being." No longer do we see the care of the patient as a burden to carry out or a duty to perform. Instead, we realize the great honor of ministering to a human being. In so doing we enter into the mystery of being human.

When patients enter the terminal phase of dying, we see them stripped of their protective mental mechanisms, the physical strength to put their best foot forward, and the constant distraction of activity, possessions, and things that must be done. Here, at the threshold of each human's second greatest transition (the greatest being the transition from darkness into light through new birth in Christ), we gain a sense of the presence of God rarely known otherwise. Everything that happens at this time has a sense of God working through us beyond our own capacity.

Paul's words come to us anew, "For you are the temple of the living God. As God said: 'I will dwell in them and walk among them. I will be their God and they will be my people'" (2 Cor. 6:16, NKJB).

Discover that Life Follows Death

As we look at our own dying, we recognize a greater depth in our own lives. We'll find new meaning to our lives as well. Jesus demonstrated this principle of life at Golgatha: there is no life without death. Had He not died on the cross, we would not have life. And Paul says, "For if you live according to the flesh you will die; but if you through the Spirit put to death the deeds of the body, you will live (Rom. 8:13, NKJB).

Dying is an important part of life. Our daily living can be seen as a series of deaths as we go through the stages of life. Yet, after each of these stages comes a new stage of life. The family can explore these death equivalents (stages) as a group and learn from each other what it means to grow old and to mature as a person.

Referring to the normal death equivalents of life on regular occasions and seeing each as a preparation for a higher plane of living brings confidence to family members that can sustain them through any death. For they will have learned to anticipate new beginnings. Even the loss of a girlfriend or boyfriend can be seen as a death equivalent and the preparation for a more mature relationship next time.

See Death as a Natural Part of Life

Furthermore, preparing the family for death can be accomplished by planning activities that will assure family members that death is a natural part of life.

I definitely believe that every family member needs to see the dying member's body when he or she finally dies. Various studies of war victims also showed the detrimental effects on a spouse, in particular, when she did not actually see her husband's dead body. Closure becomes very difficult if family members cannot visualize the loved one as dead. When circumstances prevent this, a picture can be taken of the casket, and this will help immensely.

Visits to dying grandparents, other relatives, and friends can help establish the finality of death and the naturalness of it. Commemorative funerals can relieve anxiety in children over the event of death.

Share the Grief

Open, dynamic relationships within the family on a regular basis where the lives of its members are discussed and their feelings and responses carefully regarded sets the stage for frank discussions of death and dying when these happen. The whole family should be exposed to the pain and suffering— whatever the cause—of the other family members at whatever level they can understand. Sharing the pain does not remove it, but it certainly lessens its sting and makes it bearable. If we deny and try to hide the pain of other family members, we deceive a child and rob him or her of the opportunity to learn and grow through problems. We all need to learn to keep control of our attitudes and motives even when the circumstances are out of our control.

No problem or difficulty or tragedy that happens to a family member should be excluded in order to protect someone. There may be valid reasons for softening the impact of some experiences for small children. But the norm should be that whatever happens to one person can happen to any other. So if we desire to prepare children for life, they need to be exposed to it at an age-appropriate intensity. And how wonderful it is to share difficulties with our kids when we can be around to help them go through those difficulties, ask questions, and then lead them to the resources they need—as Christ does with us.

As an illustration of this, let me tell you of my training in surgery. Our residency program was set up so that each surgical resident got the widest exposure to disease possible. We had daily sharing of cases with the group, and weekly lectures on different diseases. And we told each other in great detail the new expressions of any disease we found. Then we shared the treatment given or anticipated. In this way each resident, when graduated, would have the widest knowledge of disease possible when serving his or her own patients. Aren't you happy that your doctor had this type of training too?

Form the Family into a Support Group

To accomplish this in greater detail, organize the family into a support group for each other. Cry together, fear together, praise together, and smile together. Teach each other how to be compassionate and comforting in times of need, the purpose being to help the suffering one get in touch with his or her feelings and to deal with them adequately. We can often see positive values in a situation that the suffering person misses. Remember that these difficult times are death equivalents, and the way we help others face them sets the stage for how they will perceive and behave when they are dying.

In all situations within the family, aim to help each family member face the reality of the situations of his or her life and make the tough choices that are often required. Help family members respect the rights of others when they are trying to help rather than taking over "for the other's good." This process provides great confidence to children and adults that, whatever life has to offer, God can help them cope with it and, very possibly, transcend it.

Preserve Continuity

Preserving the family's everyday life gives a sense of continuity to the one in the difficult situation. And the constant personal contact during hard times is able to provide the continuity that the child needs for reassurance. Here our faithfulness and our continued presence supports the person throughout his or her life.

With a solid basis of continuity and trust from those they love and know best, children can develop a sense of dignity of highest human worth in themselves and each member of their family.

Show Appreciation for Life

Develop a sense of life as a gift to be lived in appreciation for the opportunity of living and sharing it with others rather than life as a right to everything the world has to offer. Help each member see his life as a project to be fashioned in his own way, to be cherished and committed to, regardless of what the circumstances of life bring.

Fan the flames of hope. Help children see opportunities for hope in everything. Even when a situation seems hopeless, hold out hope. Help them to see the dynamic nature of hope and how our greatest hope lives within our life's own development and is not dependent on outside circumstances or influences. Teach them to go to the source of hope for all humans and not to be defeated by anxiety, despair, and depression that come from the situation.

Surround with Love

And finally, to best prepare family members for death we need to provide a solid love relationship for each person in the family and make each person responsible for his or her part. The certainty that every individual is needed encourages freedom of expression and sharing of intimate emotions even when that person feels quite vulnerable.

Develop mature love relationships between each and all members of the family. These relationships should be free of manipulation, coercion, and deceit. There is a mutual respect for the dignity of the other. Each family member should not demand from the others that his or her needs be met.

Independence should be fostered, and the growth and development of each person should occur in a peaceful and harmonious atmosphere. Here no one need give up his or her identity to care for another. A deep feeling of togetherness, an attraction for one another, and a closeness of spirits should be cultivated. In this way a feeling of belonging can keep fear, isolation, and loneliness at a minimum. And through family members the person can have a strong sense of control of situations in which he or she cannot have any direct control.

Support for the Family

When a family has a lack of growth as they are going through trials and sufferings, the family may need outside assistance. A pastor, doctor, chaplain, or trained lay person may help, but professional help may be required. If so, don't hesitate to get it.

Many nursing homes and other community institutions are developing support groups for the family which can provide a lot of assistance. In Long Beach, California, for instance, a day-care center has been set up to take care of patients suffering from Alzheimer's disease. The family can take direct care of the patient on weekends, evenings, and nights, but the day-care center will provide supervision, meals, and activities during the day. This allows family members to continue working, going to school, shopping, and time to do the necessary house work. Some families can even plan day vacations which offer rest and relaxation from the constant responsibility of caring for the Alzheimer patient.

Recently, an organization called Mothers of AIDS Patients (MAP) began in San Diego. This support group meets twice weekly and helps mothers share their grief. The families of the AIDS patients learn to ease the pain caused by the disease. They address the many questions and problems that arise in families with AIDS patients. The group brainstorms—based on the experience of its members—to figure out what they can do to help each member. One needs to talk with the AIDS patient about dying. One of these mothers "was able to talk to her son about his death and it was OK with both of them when the time came. I think she feels very complete about it."[4]

These two illustrations represent the numerous support groups available to dying families. They demonstrate that modern technology does not help us as much as the support of other people.

Outlining a Person's Life

This book focuses on a person's life being a gift from God, and flowing from that premise comes our responsibility to fashion our lives into all they can be with God's help. I have called this our "life's masterpiece."

But when a family faces the death of one of its members, we need to know how to understand that member's masterpiece. How can we cast the right light on it to best portray its panorama?

Let's look at an outline for reviewing a person's life with this question in mind.

1. What kind of a person is he or she?
2. Is his or her intelligence characterized by common sense, wisdom, great education?
3. What has been the person's life orientation—
   a. practical?
   b. idealistic?
   c. motivated, committed?
   d. inspired, visionary?
   e. follower or leader?
4. What does this person model for me? What is his or her major priority? What would I say about his or her masterpiece? Did this person attain a high degree of their potential?
5. What attitudes and truths were taught to me?
6. What are this person's favorite Scriptures and songs?
7. What is the person's dying style—
   a. as he or she lived?
   b. changed by great regression?
   c. demonstrating continued maturation?
8. How did the person meet problems and difficulties in his or her life? How is death being faced?
   a. denial?
   b. anger?
   c. compromise?

d. depression?
e. in stride—working on the solution?
f. ran away?
g. negative or positive perspective?
9. How might I apply this personally?
   a. What do I see of myself in this person?
   b. What should I add to my life or subtract from it?
   c. What does this review reveal about me?

This outline only suggests significant points, and you are free to create any kind of story or account of your loved one. But I'd like to demonstrate how I used this outline in creating a narrative for my father.

My Father's Life's Masterpiece

After a year of rapid deterioration of his back bone, my father died on October 24, 1984.

Dad was a man of wisdom and insight. Not many people knew of my father, yet he was a great man—a rare and essential man. He was a man to whom many people came for insight and wisdom.

Like the Prophet Ezra in the Bible, Dad was a priest, a man who set his heart to study the Scriptures, to practice what the Bible taught, and to share the Word that he learned and practiced. Not only did he get into the Word, but the Word got into him. On Sunday he "rightly divided the Word," and on Monday he modeled it. This integrity was transparent and attracted others to him.

He never claimed to be the source of truth, but he introduced me to the source of truth, Jesus Christ. Dad was an inspiring model, an Ezra for me: he studied the Word, so I wanted to study it too. He taught me how to study and apply the Word to my life so that I might gain wisdom. He practiced the Word before me so that I might gain experience in applying the Word to my life.

Let me share some examples: (1) In any difficulty, I need to go to God about my part before confronting others about their part. (2) Never be a part of the problem; always be a part of the solution. Ask God to start the solution in you. (3) He who leads the best seems not to lead at all. (4) He taught me to love my wife by the way he daily loved my mother. (5) He taught me how to raise and love my children by the way he raised and loved me. (6) He taught me how to love and care for my patients by the way he loved and cared for his parishioners.

The integrity of Dad's life was displayed in his dying. He refused to succumb to the pain and agony of the bony deterioration of his spine and his frequently fractured ribs. In his last days, he knew His Lord intimately and he took everything to God in prayer and praise. The peace he experienced throughout his life was evident during his entire dying process. The peace Dad displayed in his dying stimulated me greatly. I have taken care of many dying patients, but I've never witnessed such peace as Dad showed. His faith and confidence in God over 79 years was verified and ratified in the last months of his dying. He loved the line from the song: "When peace like a river attendeth my way, when sorrows like sea billows roll; whatever my lot, Thou has taught me to say, 'It is well, it is well with my soul.' "

He was so stimulated by the Scriptures that even in his dying he quoted and sang Scriptures to us.

During one of the weeks before my Dad died I brought my older three teenagers back to Indiana to spend a week caring for their grandpa. Each of them stayed with friends, but each took a turn every third day spending all day with Grandma and me taking care of Grandpa.

My personal involvement that week will always count as one of the greatest and most meaningful experiences of my entire life. Just moments before we left to return to California, we all stood around Dad's bed. He was too weak to get out of bed or sit up to say good-bye. We made a circle around him and each of us prayed aloud for him. Then it was his turn. He gazed at us a few moments, then, with a loud and clear voice he burst into singing Psalm 103, "Bless the Lord, O my soul, and all that is within me. Bless his holy name!"

Throughout my life Dad always encouraged me to be the best person I could be. He modeled and lived that type of victorious life. And in his dying he has encouraged me to trust God in my dying. For he demonstrated that in our circumstance of greatest weakness and loss, Christ offers his great strength and comfort. No wonder Dad's gravestone says, "Encourager."

Notes

1 Marvin Bryan, "1988, the Year of the Data Base," *Personal Computing*, Jan. 1988, p. 100.
2 Dick Walt, "Financing Longterm Care for the Elderly," *American Medical News*, January 15, 1988, p. 27.
3 Melvin J. Krant, *Dying and Dignity* (Springfield, Illinois: Charles C. Thomas Publisher, 1974), p. 34.
4 Sari Staver, *American Medical News*, Jan. 22/29, 1988, p. 3.

CHAPTER THIRTEEN

Models of Others Who Have Gone Before

This book has been concerned with dying, not just death. Dying is a process. What have we learned about the Christian perspective of dying? I believe it can be summarized in the following principles.

1. God made the dying process a universal part of every life, even the lower animals and plants.

2. Therefore, the dying process has meaning and purpose for the individual person and the whole of the human race. It is the way of nature for everyone, not some abnormal circumstance. It brings together the whole of life. To die well requires the best of what we have become throughout life. So, in a real sense, the dying process is not an indignity in itself, since it is a part of life. Dying is to be accepted and expected by everyone. The dying process cannot be contrasted with the rest of life to say that it is thereby dehumanizing. It has been set as the final limit of our earthly existence and, therefore, is a genuine expression of our humanness.

3. In fact, for the Christian, dying is a part of one's witness to the world of God's presence and resource that goes beyond the dying process.

4. Many of us have had near-death experiences or death equivalents that have prepared us intellectually for our own

death. But for the Christian, dying ultimately provides a unique experience with God that cannot be obtained any other way. As Paul said, it is designed so that we will depend on God and not self. And Peter says that our faith is to be proved genuine and result in praise, glory, and honor when Jesus Christ is revealed. Christ is Lord of the dying process too.

5. God is the God of compassion and all comfort, even in the dying process, and that is sufficient comfort for any dying process.

6. Human dignity lies in transcending the circumstances of life, in transcending creation, by the indwelling Creator.

7. Suicide is wrong not just because God is supposed to decide when death is to come to a person, but because it is an outright statement that God is not sufficient for the problems of life. In other words, it proclaims that God made a mistake in designing the world, or that He is not sovereign or master of it all. It is putting the creature before the Creator, which is the basis of sin.

Following the Glory Road

When we must face any difficult challenge, it is helpful to see how others have met a similar trial. Sometimes we are informed by their views, sometimes inspired by their courage, and often reassured by their (and our) humanness.

So it is with the great transition from this life to the next. It's not macabre curiosity to ask, "How did he or she die?" meaning not so much what was the cause of death as the *way* the person faced death. Indeed, in our modern, sanitized world, many people have never seen a person die except on TV, where it is often made both unrealistic and commonplace in a detached sort of way.

As in everything, Christ is the supreme example for the Christian. Consider these aspects of how He faced death.

- It was a hard trial for Him. He was not exempt just because He was certain of the hereafter.

- Christ's great struggle in prayer on the Mount of Olives illustrates that He faced the real temptation to avoid His "cup of suffering," just as some of us wonder whether we can't avoid the dying process and end it all quickly.
- Jesus said He could have called on 12 legions of angels to deliver Him, if that had been right.
- When Peter actually attempted to protect Him, Christ rebuked him, asking, "Shall I not drink the cup the Father has given me?" (John 18:11)
- He announced His death with the words, "It is finished," underlining for us that there is real purpose right up through the last moment.

With Christ as their model, how have other believers approached the end of their lives, especially when they had some choices they could make? Here are a few recent models I feel honored to recommend.

MOTHER
"Happiness First"[1]
By Ruth Graham

We felt that keeping Mother as happy as possible after Daddy died was more important than keeping her well. We let her do exactly what she wanted, whether it was good for her or not.

I've seen too many old people whose lives were made miserable because of bossy children.

When she was ready, we moved her up to live with us. We had prepared the downstairs guest room years before with this in mind, putting in a bay window to add light. It had its own little fireplace and private bath.

But after a few weeks, we found that what Bill and I needed was what Mother did not need. We need quiet and privacy. Mother needed people.

When she asked if she could move back to her house, we said, "Whatever makes you happiest."

So we located a housekeeper and a companion and moved her back.

Friends and neighbors dropped in constantly. One day a group of students from the college came and gathered about her, sitting on whatever was available, spilling onto the floor. One had a guitar, and they sang hymns and choruses for her till the house bulged with music, and Mother knew she was surrounded by love.

Then she had a final stroke. I was in Mequon recovering from my fall when word reached us that Mother was in the hospital.

GiGi flew home with me. Rosa came, too, and Clayton from Dallas. We found Mother helpless and furious. Tubes were extending from everywhere. Her rings had been forcibly removed, and when the nurse tried to remove her partials as well, Mother, with her old spunk, snapped at her. Although she was unable to speak, I could read the anger and frustration in her eyes. This might be a postponement of death for her, but it was certainly not a prolongation of life.

So I asked the doctor who had cared for her and Daddy for so long, if we could take her home. She might not live as long, but she would die happily.

"If all you children agree," he replied, "you have my permission."

Rosa rode in the ambulance with her. She said Mother looked worried till they passed through the arched stone Montreat Gate. Then her face lit up. In her slightly confused state, she may have thought we were taking her to a nursing home (a thing she dreaded).

It was a joy to see her settled comfortably in her own bed, in her loved and familiar surroundings. Rosa was able to give her the necessary shots to keep her comfortable.

Mother, who all her life had loved music, who used to play the piano and sing like a bird, now asked only for "The King Is Coming."

Realizing that when a person is facing death and knows it, most music—even many hymns—has no appeal, we gathered a great pile of Christian records and marked every hymn that would speak to the dying. Taking them to our Christian radio station, we had them lift those particular hymns onto cassette tapes. Mother had a simple cassette recorder she was able to work, and she listened to those grand old hymns by the hour.

Then, quietly, on November 7, 1974, she joined Daddy.

CYNTHIA KANE
"The Best Years of My Life"

In order to explain why my cancer experience has meant so much to me, I have to go back 20 years. My husband was a minister, and a marvelous man. We had a wonderful marriage with two fine sons. I felt that I could look the world over without finding a better Christian than he was. And that made our home a happy one. Suddenly, he got cancer. Then I had to face myself full force, and that was the starting of a different feeling of life for me.

I felt that I could not give him up. I just couldn't do it. But John said to me, "Let's pray that God will have *His* way, for neither of us wants to go against God's will." John didn't fear death: "I can't possibly lose. If I die and go to heaven, I gain Christ and eternity. If God wants me to live here on earth, that would be fine, because He would have plans for my life."

So, we began to pray together. However, right in the middle, he stopped and said, "Hon, you're not praying with faith, are you?" I replied that I didn't know. He continued, "You're praying for God's will, but at the same time you're praying that His will might be your will, that you won't have to give me up."

Our lives had been molded together for 40 years, and I had to admit that I just couldn't give him up.

So I left the house and drove to a field over which the sun was setting. I got out of the car and walked into the sunset and prayed like I had never prayed before. The rays of the sun glistened and inspired my heart to such an extent that I was lifted in spirit by its beauty. It made me feel as if I were walking into heaven.

I asked God to help me say yes to His will. And you know, I felt as if pounds of weight were rolling off me. I almost looked around me to see what the load had been. The grace that God gave me then, took me through the rest of John's illness, his death, and my grief.

Five years ago I discovered that I had cancer. Since then, it has spread to all the bones of my body as well as my lung and chest. I have not been able to go many places or do for others or even myself. But these have been the best five years of my life. When a friend asked me how I could say such a thing in the midst of all the pain, I answered that I see death, now, as the conclusion of my journey through life. I know I am right with God, so death is no problem; there is no fear. I feel that death can be beautiful. I told her that there is so much of life that I didn't get to experience when I was so busy with "activities." My house, my car, going from here to there, and getting *things* all seem so trivial.

What's important now is worship. I've had experiences of worship like I've never had before. And lots of times, it is just by myself. I have had more time to search my inner self. When I was in the nursing home, I saw anew the beauty of the trees and flowers and the sunsets—all those marvelous things that only God could design. When I got home, I saw the beauty of spring in my own trees and flowers. It seems as if there's something more of God here.

I've enjoyed the trees and blossoms, but the thing above all else that thrills me is the new beauty of people that I had missed before. I used to get so aggravated with some people when they did stupid things. But now I don't. I can see something else in them besides errors. I'm not looking for errors anymore, I'm looking for goodness, and that helps me be much more tolerant and patient.

When I was so active I never took time to grow. Instead of growing inwardly, I pursued good works. I often didn't take time to look at myself as I really was. It's been beautiful to learn to love people more. I've learned to love my family more, if that were possible. I thought I loved them as much as any person could love. In the hospital, I've met people who unknowingly passed something on to me that has helped me build a deeper life. I see so much of God everywhere I look.

If my life can be a blessing to anyone, I want to live. But I'm ready to die anytime He comes to take me. I'm not striving to live, I don't pray to live. I only pray for the strength to be able to do something worthwhile while I'm alive.

When I think of my life before my cancer, I didn't seem to need God very much. I would just go on my own way depending on myself so much. Sometimes I'd even forget to pray. Now I've learned how to trust Him. Now when I come to where I really need Him, He's there. God is so much more a real person than He ever was before.

The thing that started this whole new way of life for me, as I mentioned before, was John's dying and that little walk in the country where I met God. The strength and the grace that He gave me then, when I committed myself to His will, made a different person of me.

It was my privilege to be Cynthia Kane's doctor during her six-year bout with cancer. She endured great pain. The cobalt treatments she received caused vomiting, fatigue, hoarseness, and shortness of breath. Toward the end, her right arm shook uncontrollably, and that depressed her whenever she thought about it. But she said that prayer, more than anything, helped her rise above that depression.

As Victor Frankl said: "To live is to suffer, and to survive is to find meaning in that suffering." Cynthia died in triumph on July 26, 1980, at the age of 80.

CORRIE TEN BOOM
"Free at Last"

Corrie ten Boom died over a long drawn-out period of deterioration caused by several strokes, which robbed her of her verbal and writing abilities to communicate. This five-year process was the kind that makes many people say, "Why? Why should anyone have to endure that kind of prolonged suffering? Wouldn't it be so much more merciful to end her suffering?"

Corrie often talked about heaven and her longing to be there. But she didn't mention her own dying much and only in general terms: "Bury me in the back garden—this body is only my shell. I myself will be more alive than I have ever been."[2]

In her book, *Tramp for the Lord,* Corrie did discuss death as she had faced it in a Nazi concentration camp during World War II: "When you are dying—when you stand at the gate of eternity—you see things from a different perspective than when you think you may live a long time. I had been standing at that gate for many months, living in Barracks 28 in the shadow of the crematorium. Every time I saw the smoke pouring from the hideous smokestacks I knew it was the remains of some poor woman who had been with me in Ravensbruck. I often asked myself, 'When will it be my time to be killed or die?'

"But I was not afraid. Following [my sister] Betsie's death, God's presence was even more real. Even though I was looking into the valley of the shadow of death, I was not afraid. It is here that Jesus comes the closest, taking our hand, and leading us through."[3]

A week after Betsie's death in Ravensbruck, where 96,000 women died, Corrie took her place in the ranks of women prisoners standing together in the icy cold of the early morning roll call, which lasted three hours. But instead of calling her "Prisoner 66730," her own name was called, and she was told to stand to the side with some other prisoners. Thinking they had received a death sentence, Corrie prayed: "Perhaps I'll see you face-to-face, like Betsie does now, Lord. Let it not be too cruel a killing. Not gas, Lord, not hanging, I prefer shooting. It is so quick. You see something, you hear something, and it is finished . . . Lord, this is perhaps the last chance I will have to bring someone to You before I arrive in heaven. Use me, Lord. Give me all the love and wisdom I need."[4] And the Lord did use Corrie to lead a young girl standing next to her to Him.

But instead of a death sentence, Corrie and the other women who had been singled out were given a "Certificate of Discharge" and released from the prison camp. "I was free," recalled Corrie, "and flooding through my mind were the words of Jesus to the church at Philadelphia: 'Behold, I have set before thee an open door, and no man can shut it.' "[5]

In the spring of 1979 Corrie complained about a headache for several days. Then she had a major stroke. She no longer had the ability to speak and understand, nor could she read, write, interpret gestures, or make meaningful signs to those around her.

One night her friend, Pamela Rosewella, was leaving the hospital when she recalled a statement Corrie had repeated often, "Child, it is not so much what happens, but how we take it that is important. God is watching to see whether we allow the problems to defeat us, or whether we will go through them in His strength, being made stronger for the next problem and ultimately for the final end battle."[6]

Corrie went home but had another stroke, and finally a third in the autumn of 1980, from which she never got up. Her doctor diagnosed pneumonia. He said it was time to make a decision: if she were admitted to the hospital, she would have to undergo the standard treatment of antibiotics, respirator, and so forth. Those closest to her decided to keep her at home, receiving care from those who knew her best.

Corrie's ministry took on new significance when she lost her verbal and writing skills. "She was able to show all who knew her in the last years of her life that He is always, always, always with us," relates biographer Carole C. Carlson.

"The visitors who left Corrie's bedside saw a peace that 'passes all understanding.' Many said that if she could be joyful in the Lord in her circumstances, then they surely could be in theirs.

"Pam [Rosewella] said, 'I had always seen the Lord Jesus in

her, but now in her present physical weakness, I see Him so much more clearly. She is always pointing Lotte and me to Him—sometimes literally with her hand as she points to heaven and says with a radiant face, 'I cannot . . . but He . . . He can.' "

"As the months stretched into years and the great communicator remained mute, her body gradually becoming weaker as age and successive strokes took their toll, the lessons to be learned from this last phase of her long life became clearer. Through her example and the loving care of those who surrounded her, we were able to see God's view of human life. She was making an important statement in this humanistic world: that however limited physical circumstances may be, human life is made in the image of God, is precious and worth living."[7]

Pamela Rosewella tells of her final visit with this inspiring woman: "We sang to her a little of two Dutch hymns, one about the lovely name of Jesus and the other, "Praise God with Waves of Joy." We told her that we loved her, but what was much more important, that nothing could separate her from the love of God in Jesus Christ. She opened her eyes and we knew that she had understood. Later that night she became completely unconscious and her limbs were very cold. Then I heard a sound from Corrie's bedroom. Running to her side I saw that Corrie's breathing pattern had changed. Three of us stood there as Corrie breathed for the last time and very peacefully went to the Lord Jesus. There were no heavenly revelations. The room was quiet and peaceful just before she left us. It was quiet and peaceful after she left us. It was three minutes to eleven in the evening of her birthday, April 15, 1983, ninety-one years to the day of her birth and exactly on time.[8]

JOSEPH T. BAYLY
by Nathan Bayly

In the long line of hospital carts in a stark corridor, Joe Bayly waited and thought: "The surgery will not be very serious, there is little risk, but I am equally at peace, as far as I can plumb the depths of my heart, with either prospect. I wonder how many others in the long white line have this hope. How would I feel, approaching the radical surgical procedures some of them face, without it? Would I have their courage?"[9]

Joe later faced those questions, but not without hope. For his faith had blossomed more than half a century earlier and continued to grow. And so he faced death with the same faith as he had lived life. He considered death an event—not an end—and was as eager to complete his dying process when the time came as he was any other experience of life. Thus, he wrote:

Lord
if anything happens
if you come for me
keep them from interfering
desperately trying
to tug me
from your grasp.
If I'm far
across the river
where you own the shore
and all beyond
don't let them
bring me back
prolonging death
not life
delaying life
that never crosses
the unreturning river
again.[10]

But God did not call Joe home from that vein-stripping surgery for which he waited in the hospital corridor. There was yet more work for him to do.

Due to his acceptance of the directorship of the Christian

Medical Society while continuing as the vice president of David C. Cook Publishing Co., his work load was greatly increased. He carried on the ministry he felt God had given him of traveling to teach, preach, and speak wherever and whenever he was free to do so. And he remained prolific, writing articles for a variety of magazines, including *Eternity,* narrating a weekly spot about his opinions on religion in America for the UPI, and authoring several books.

Joe was never one to shy from speaking the truth. An example was his bold predictions in his futuristic novel *Winterflight.* There he painted the bleakness that will likely come to our society from its high-tech medical trends if we do not reestablish our moral and ethical base.

On a trip to Mexico City for a CMS conference, Joe passed out on the plane, yet he presented his address at the conference before spending the next week in the hospital due to that heart incident.

From that time on, his heart became more of a problem, hindering his progress in a few areas, goading him on with increased urgency in others. Due to the medication for his heart, Joe began to perceive a slow loss of mental acuity and memory.

Perhaps his most treasured and enjoyed skill was creativity, upon which he relied for his writing. And as he began to notice a loss of sharpness, he felt God was showing him that his most effective ministry lay in preaching and speaking; therefore, he continued to travel at a wearing schedule, even for someone in good health.

Joe's family was keenly aware of the symptoms of illness he was unable to hide: shortness of breath that eventually prevented him from walking a hundred paces across Illinois' flat land without stopping, spells of crossness arising from his pain, continuing weariness, and depression.

Though the family urged, he was unwilling to become dependent on frequent visits to the doctor, relying instead on regular checkups at Mayo Clinic in Rochester, Minnesota.

After experiencing a massive heart attack in upstate Michigan without realizing what was happening, he agreed with his doctor that an angiogram was needed to determine the condition of his heart. The test was scheduled for July 1986, following a family vacation at the Jersey shore. The vacation culminated in a time of prayer during which the family gathered around Joe, laid their hands on him, and committed him to God's care.

Feeling the angiogram at Mayo would be routine, Joe wanted no family with him. Only when the results indicated he needed immediate surgery to complete four bypasses did he ask his wife, Mary Lou, to join him.

Joe was anticipating the prospect of renewed health after the surgery. Because of good reports beforehand, only one of the four children—the oldest son Timothy and his wife Mary Lee who lived in nearby Wisconsin—joined Mary Lou at the hospital.

The bypass surgery was complicated by the need to replace a valve, but all went smoothly. Joe was removed from the heart/lung machine in the recovery room without a problem. He was then transferred to the ICU. There his heart became uncontrollable, and God honored his wish not to remain on earth when heaven beckoned. He died July 16, 1986.

His legacy might best be found in the September '86 column of his popular, "Out of My Mind," that regularly enlivened *Eternity* magazine. Just before his death Joe wrote a farewell column ending his 25-year relationship with the magazine after the publication had changed hands. In it he said: "Mary Lou and I . . . know that both by His severity and by His goodness God has shown consistent faithfulness. God is good. He is worthy of all trust and all glory. Amen."

FRANCIS SCHAEFFER
"Till Death Do Us Part"[11]
by Edith Schaeffer

Fran came across the Atlantic Ocean from L'Abri, Switzerland, in December 1983 for cancer treatment at the Mayo Clinic in

Rochester, Minnesota. He was very ill, and the flight was a difficult one. On the way from the airport to the hospital, the doctors in the ambulance were reporting by walkie-talkie his pulse beat, blood pressure, and rate of breathing, all of which were rather alarming. When we finally got to the hospital, a doctor told me he doubted Fran would live through the night. I told him I would call upon God and ask Him to be the one to make that judgment.

The next morning, Fran was better. He opened his eyes and said to me, "Edith, would you be willing to buy a house near the hospital so I don't ever have to cross the ocean again, and so I could go home and have my things around me?" Of course I said I would, believing that was part of what I had promised in my marriage vows when I said, "For better or worse . . . till death do us part."

That evening, I passed a house with a "For Sale" sign in the lawn, and within a week I was signing the papers. A month later, I was back at L'Abri, packing all the possessions of our married life into 269 boxes. It was another five weeks until those boxes reached Rochester. During that time, Fran was in and out of the hospital and on two speaking tours. He was only in the newly furnished house two days before he returned to the hospital for the last time.

On Easter Day, six doctors called me into a room, and the leading consultant said, "He is dying of cancer. Do you want him placed in intensive care on machines? Once a person is on machines, I would never pull the plug. I need to know what your viewpoint is."

Many thoughts went through my head. I had for years talked with my husband about the preciousness of life, of the fact that even five minutes can make a difference if something needs to be said or needs to be done. We did not believe in putting a chain around our necks with a living will, because doctors and ambulance aids can make terrible mistakes. They could find that tag and push that person aside and take care of someone else, when the one with the living will could have lived for another five years if given oxygen at the right time.

But there is no point in prolonging death. It is a fine line; it is not an absolute one-two-three process. There are differences from person to person, and it requires great wisdom. Based on these thoughts, I told the doctor, "My feeling right now is that above all things, Fran wants to be with me. I haven't left him at all. I believe when my husband leaves his body, he will be with the Lord. I don't want him to leave me until he's with the Lord. Therefore, I am sure he would want to go to the house he asked me to buy and be there for the time he has left."

The doctors got the most relieved looks on their faces. One of them said, "I just wish more people would do things this way. That's the best kind of care at this time. That's the most helpful thing."

Soon Fran was home, in a bed facing four big panels of glass looking out on a deck with grass around it and trees with the first leaves of spring. The L'Abri workers went out and bought pots of geraniums so there would be an instant garden all around the window. All the things Fran loved in Switzerland were around him, just as he asked.

Music flooded the room. One after another, we played his favorite records: Beethoven, Bach, Schubert, and Handel. Ten days later, on May 15, 1984, with the music of Handel's *Messiah* still in the air, Fran breathed his last breath.

And He shall reign forever and ever . . .
King of kings and Lord of lords . . .
Hallelujah, hallelujah.[12]

Notes

[1] Ruth Graham, *It's My Turn* (Old Tappan, New Jersey: Fleming H. Revell Co., 1982), pp. 180–181. Used by permission.
[2] Pamela Rosewella, *The Five Silent Years* (Grand Rapids, Michigan: Zondervan, 1986,), p. 79.
[3] Corrie ten Boom, *Tramp for the Lord* (Fort Washington, Pennsylvania: Christian Literature Crusade, 1974), p. 23.
[4] Ibid., pp. 19–24.
[5] Ibid.
[6] Rosewella, p. 109–110.

[7] Carole C. Carlson, *Corrie ten Boom: Her Life and Her Faith* (Old Tappan, New Jersey: Fleming H. Revell, Co., 1983) pp. 219–221.

[8] Rosewella, p. 184

[9] Joseph Bayly, *Heaven* (Elgin, Illinois: David C. Cook Pub. Co., 1977), p. 6. Used by permission of David C. Cook Pub. Co.

[10] Joseph Bayly, "A Psalm On Viewing the River," *Psalms of My Life*, (Elgin, Illinois: David C. Cook Pub. Co., 1987 by estate of Joseph Bayly), p. 36. Used by permission of David C. Cook Pub. Co.

[11] Edith Schaeffer, "Till Death Do Us Part," *Christianity Today*, March 6, 1987, p. 20. Used by permission of the author.

[12] George Frideric Handel, from the *Messiah*, 1742.

Understanding Brain Death

The old definition of brain death served medicine and society well when we could only accurately diagnose whole brain death. This means death of the cerebral cortex (including the neocortex), midbrain and brain stem. That traditional definition of death with total cessation of breathing and pulse in an unconscious person, however, today has become inadequate. As Nobel Prize winner Dr. Gerald M. Edelman states, "In the past 10 years, we have learned more about the brain than in all of history."[1]

Previously, people thought the whole brain died as a unit. If any sign of life remained, the patient was a living human being. Now we can diagnosis the death of the components of the brain and at what stage of dying a person is no longer a living human being. This occurs, for example, when the surviving brain stem maintains the bodily functions but the dying cerebral cortex fails to exhibit human personality—the state of the *living corpse.*

Therefore, when the cerebrum dies (quits functioning), the human person no longer exists. The body will never move, respond or interact with anything or anyone. The old term "suspended animation" applies here, for all the potential for unique human ability and maturity as well as the very spirit, enthusiasm, vibrancy and zest of human life no longer remains. Why? Because the lower portions of the brain have no functions which differentiate the human being from the rest of the animal kingdom. As an example, the brain stem contains the center for the control of pulse and blood pressure. Yet the control of circulation differs little from the heart's pumping of blood. The cerebral cortex, in contrast, cannot regulate the pulse or the blood pressure. But it does decide those activities which give meaning and purpose to the pulse and blood pressure.

By saying this, I do not mean that we should be concerned about only the cerebral cortex. I certainly do want to stress the unity of the whole person (body, mind, and soul). My point here, though, focuses on the hierarchy of these. For instance, consider this common problem. A business executive of a company may be required to travel across the country to carry out the corporation's business. To value transportation, lodging,

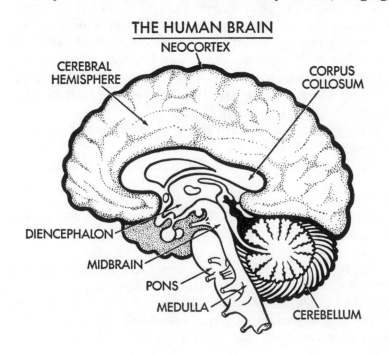

THE HUMAN BRAIN

NEOCORTEX

CEREBRAL HEMISPHERE

CORPUS COLLOSUM

DIENCEPHALON

MIDBRAIN

PONS

MEDULLA

CEREBELLUM

meals, etc. as equivalent to the accomplishing of the corporation's goals degrades the job and is inaccurate. No matter how far the corporate executive travels he does not accomplish his role for the company unless he completes the corporation's business. With the brain it is the cerebral cortex and especially its neocortex that performs the human's transactions.

To gain a better understanding of these statements of brain death, let us look at a picture of the human brain and its parts.

The human brain has three major divisions: forebrain, midbrain and the hindbrain, which lie in that order from the top of the cranial cavity to its base. The functions of the brain though can be generally divided into those functions which result in production of personality and those concerned with maintaining the physical body in service of the personality.

The Parts of the Brain Concerned with Personality

The forebrain contains most of the brain tissue which lies within the skull and forms the two *cerebral hemispheres.* Each hemisphere contains five lobes: frontal, temporal, parietal, and occipital. The fifth lobe, the limbic (smell), consists of the middle surface of the cerebrum, where the hemispheres meet each other. The deeper portion is white matter. The *corpus callosum* connects the two hemispheres together by a thick band of white matter.

- *The cerebral cortex*—On the surface of the cerebral hemispheres lies a thin layer (about 3–4mm. thick) called the cerebral cortex or gray matter. It folds into gyri with about two-thirds of its area buried in the depths of the fissures of the cerebral hemispheres. Customarily the cortex (pallium) is separated into the olfactory cortex because it occurred with the early vertebrate animals, and the non-olfactory younger cortex (neopallium) called the neocortex.[2]
- *The neocortex* represents the most highly developed tissue of all living matter and achieves the highest mental functions which occur only in the human being. It also exe-

cutes general movements, visceral functions, perception, and behavioral reactions. Only the neocortex has the ability to associate and integrate these functions.

Let's pause here a moment and clarify this further. The original (as found in the lesser animals) cerebral cortex lies in the middle, lower area of the front of the brain. And the neocortex continues from there to cover the entire cerebral hemispheres. In the lower vertebrates, most of the cerebral cortex is taken up mainly by the olfactory (smell) portion of the brain. In man, the exuberant growth of the cortex not involved in olfaction and covering the rest of the brain is called the neocortex, which contains the uniquely human characteristics.[3] Most people use the terms cerebral cortex and neocortex interchangeably since the cerebral cortex of mankind is understood as being almost totally neocortex.

The Parts of the Brain Concerned with Bodily Functions

The diencephalon lies under the cerebrum and contains the hypothalamus which controls body temperature, hunger, and thirst, and the pituitary gland—seat of emotions, such as fear and anger (but the neocortex interprets these). The *subthalamus* acts as a crossroad between the basal ganglia and plays an important part in coordinating movements. The *thalamus* relays sensory impulses to the surface of the cerebrum and from one part of the brain to another. It helps coordinate sensory messages and helps regulate the activity of the brain. Although the diencephalon rests at the bottom of the forebrain, most people consider it as part of the brain stem rather than the cerebrum. For our considerations it functions as a part of the brain stem since it does not contain the same tissue or function as the neocortex.

The midbrain or mesencephalon is the short portion of the brain stem lying between the cerebral hemispheres and the pons, which joins the medulla oblongata. The midbrain controls movements of the eyes and of other parts of the body. It also contains an important part of the reticular system.

The hindbrain: This stemlike portion of the brain connects the cerebral hemispheres with the spinal cord and contains the pons and the medulla oblongata.

- *The pons* makes up the middle part of the brain stem and acts as a relay station between the cerebrum and the cerebellum. It holds an important part of the reticular system, which controls the overall degree of central nervous system activity, including wakefulness, attentiveness, and sleep.[4]

- *The cerebellum,* the second largest portion of the brain, sits behind the pons and contains the center of muscular coordination.

- *The medulla oblongata* forms the lower part of the brain stem and connects the pons to the spinal cord. Bundles of nerve fibers that connect other parts of the brain pass through the medulla. Its nerve centers control swallowing, breathing, heartbeat, blood flow, muscle tone and posture, and movement of the stomach and intestines. It connects with the organ of balance in the ears.[5]

A Holy Place to Stand

To place this functional analysis of the brain in familiar terms, come to the operating room with me. There you'll capture the practical significance of our discussion more completely.

The other day a neurosurgeon called me to help him operate on a man. The patient had high blood pressure and was taking a medication to thin his blood for another reason. Five days ago he suddenly suffered a stroke when one of his cerebral arteries began leaking blood into his cerebral cortex. As blood leaked out of the cracked artery, it put pressure on the vital centers. A support system sustained his life for several days. However, now was the critical time to operate: blood pressure controlled, blood thinners removed, and the bleeding stopped. In the operating room we opened the skull, placed a needle on the substance of the neocortex, and slid the needle through the nerve fibers into the offending pool of blood. Aspiration immediately produced blood. Suddenly we could see the swollen, pale-blue neocortex begin to shrink and develop the normal pink color. Instantly that uniquely living human tissue, which houses the personality, began the typical, pulsating motions of vital brain tissue by responding to every heartbeat. The operation was successful!

Those mechanical features of the operation were dramatic. Yet, they cannot compare to deep feelings that stirred within my neocortex as we saw, touched, and operated upon the patient's brain. Simply the thought of working on a person's neocortex both excited and frightened me. For no other tissues of the entire body so deeply and strikingly contain the essence of a human being. Every other tissue has a specific function and contribution to the well-being of the whole person but if destroyed or its match "tissue" function replaced, the patient remains a human being. However, the neocortex remains unmatched and singular for each person.

The sight of his neocortex was breathtaking. How awesome, how inspiring, how majestic and yet mysterious! I could see that man as no one else had ever seen him. Usually we see only the skin and hair covering the head. But now I saw the very tissue inside of which the human drama takes place.

A deep sense of reverence swept over me. I recognized that I was standing in a holy place. For the Bible says, "For the Lord searches every heart and understands every motive behind the thoughts" (1 Chron. 28:9). And there I was looking at the essence of another human, a very privileged position for any human being. My neocortex began thinking and wondering, "Who is this man, what type of a person will I find if the operation is successful? On what does he base his life? What does he understand as the purpose of his life? Does he know his Creator, the one who made this brain tissue that I'm examining?"

Imagine, a human being: the pinnacle of God's creation! Envision me looking at the inner sanctum of God's highest creation. The Bible says, "When I consider Your heavens, the work of Your fingers, the moon and the stars, which You have set in place, what is man that You are mindful of him, the son of man that You care for him? You made him a little lower than the heavenly beings and crowned him with glory and honor. You made him ruler over the works of your hands; You put everything under his feet: all flocks and herds, and the beasts of the field, the birds of the air, and the fish of the sea, all that swim the paths of the seas. O Lord, our Lord, how majestic is Your name in all the earth!" (Psalm 8:3-9).

An authentic person lay on the operating table before me—not an imitation, a robot, or anything humanity could ever duplicate. Dr. Gerald M. Edelman compares the computer with the human brain. He states, "No computer could begin to deal with the variation in the world, and no computer could work if it contained connections like the enormously variable nerve-cell connections that make up the brain. The structure of the brain is not predetermined for each individual. The crucially important cell-to-cell connections in the brain are far too numerous and variable to be specified in detail by a person's genetic blueprint. So the question is how a variable brain deals with an infinitely complex, unlabeled world to make sense of things?"[6]

Add to this complexity of the human brain the variations in a person's thinking and attitudes that occur in the natural processes of aging and maturing. Then consider those single events which bring about life-changing modifications. For example, as a Christian, I recalled the dramatic and thorough change that could occur in my neocortex when I confess my sin to God and He forgives me. In no other tissues of the body could such a transformation take place. It involved a radical change in my whole understanding of life by giving me new purpose and meaning. If someone had looked at my neocortex, he or she would not have noticed any change. But inwardly, as the Bible says of every person who has been reunited to God, "Therefore, if anyone is in Christ, he is a new creation; the old has gone, the new has come!" (2 Cor. 5:17) This is why that operating room was holy ground.

Notes

[1] David Hellerstein, M.D., "Making Waves—Memory," *The Orange County Register*, June 8, 1988, sec. K.

[2] Charles Mayo Goss, A.B., M.D., *Gray's Anatomy of the Human Body* (Philadelphia: Lea and Febiger, 1973), p. 842.

[3] Ibid., p. 859

[4] *Dorland's Illustrated Medical Dictionary*, 25th ed. (Philadelphia: W.B. Saunders, 1974), p. 1238.

[5] Raymond D. Adams and Maurice Victor, M.D., *Principles of Neurology* (New York: McGraw-Hill Book Company, 1985), pp. 4–45.

[6] Hellerstein.

INDEX